REVERSING TYPE 2 DIABETES

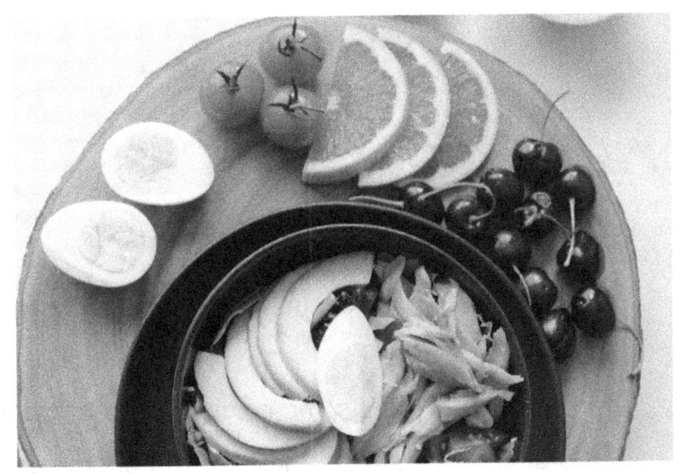

Practical Steps to Reclaiming your Health

Karla Mayer

TABLE OF CONTENT

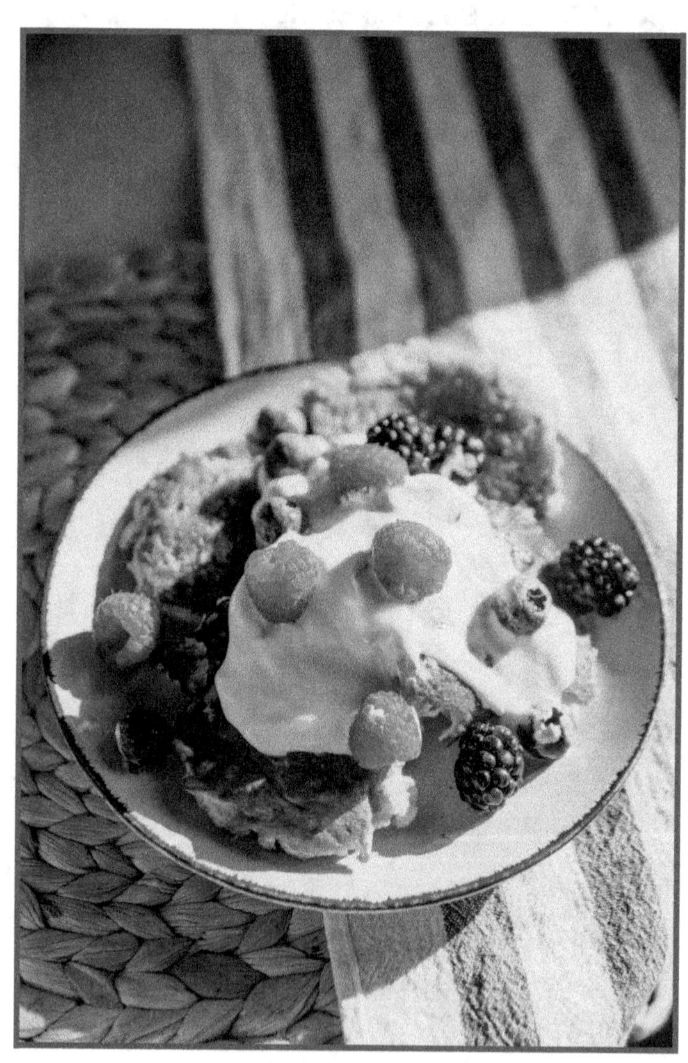

INTRODUCTION

Type 2 diabetes is a chronic condition that affects the way the body processes blood sugar, leading to high blood sugar levels. It is a serious condition that can cause a range of health problems, including heart disease, nerve damage, and kidney damage. While there is no cure for type 2 diabetes, it can be managed through lifestyle changes and medication.

Reversing type 2 diabetes refers to the process of returning the body to a state of normal blood sugar control. This can be achieved through a combination of lifestyle changes, such as diet and exercise, and medication. The goal of reversing type 2 diabetes is to improve overall health and reduce the risk of complications associated with the condition.

This page provides a comprehensive introduction to reversing type 2 diabetes, including the causes and risk factors, the benefits of reversing the condition, and the various methods for achieving this goal. We will also discuss the challenges and potential drawbacks of reversing type 2 diabetes, as well as the role of healthcare professionals in supporting individuals in their journey to reverse the condition.

By the end of this page, you will have a clear understanding of what type 2 diabetes is, how it can be reversed, and the steps you can take to improve your health and well-being.

CHAPTER ONE
Understanding Type 2 Diabetes

Type 2 diabetes is a chronic metabolic disorder characterized by the body's inability to effectively use insulin or to produce enough insulin to regulate blood sugar levels adequately. Insulin is a hormone produced by the pancreas, and it plays a crucial role in helping cells absorb glucose (sugar) from the bloodstream for energy. In individuals with type 2 diabetes, this insulin function is impaired, leading to elevated levels of blood glucose.

Understanding the complexities of type 2 diabetes is essential for those affected, as it empowers them to make informed decisions regarding lifestyle changes, medication adherence, and overall self-care to effectively manage and, in some cases, reverse the condition.

Key Factors Contributing To Type 2 Diabetes

Diabetes type 2 is a complicated illness that is impacted by a number of environmental, lifestyle, and genetic variables Several key factors contribute to the development of type 2 diabetes:

Insulin Resistance: This is a core feature of type 2 diabetes. A hormone called insulin facilitates cells' absorption of glucose from the blood. In type 2 diabetes, cells become resistant to the effects of insulin, leading to elevated blood sugar levels.

Genetics: A family history of diabetes can increase an individual's risk. Certain genes may predispose individuals to insulin resistance and impaired glucose metabolism.

Obesity: Excess body weight, particularly abdominal or visceral fat, is a significant risk factor for type 2 diabetes. Obesity contributes to insulin resistance and inflammation.

Physical Inactivity: A higher risk of type 2 diabetes is linked to a lack of consistent physical activity. Exercise helps control weight, improve insulin sensitivity, and regulate blood sugar levels.

Unhealthy Diet: Diets heavy in sugar, saturated fats, and processed carbs can exacerbate insulin resistance and obesity.. A poor diet can also lead to the development of metabolic syndrome, a cluster of conditions that increases diabetes risk.

Age: After the age of 45, there is an increased chance of type 2 diabetes. Aging is associated with a decline in metabolic function and increased likelihood of weight gain.

Ethnicity: Certain ethnic groups, such as African Americans, Hispanics, Native Americans, and Asians, have a higher predisposition to developing type 2 diabetes.

Gestational Diabetes: Type 2 diabetes is more likely to occur in later life in women who had gestational diabetes during their pregnancies.

Hormonal Factors: Conditions such as polycystic ovary syndrome (PCOS) and hormonal disorders can contribute to insulin resistance and an increased risk of type 2 diabetes.

Sleep Disorders: Poor sleep quality and insufficient sleep have been linked to an increased risk of type 2 diabetes. Sleep deprivation can affect insulin sensitivity and glucose metabolism.

Environmental Factors: Exposure to certain environmental toxins and pollutants may contribute to the development of type 2 diabetes.

It's important to note that these factors often interact, and the risk of type 2 diabetes is influenced by a combination of genetic and lifestyle elements. Making positive lifestyle changes, such as maintaining a healthy weight, engaging in regular physical activity, and adopting a balanced diet, can significantly reduce the risk of developing type 2 diabetes.

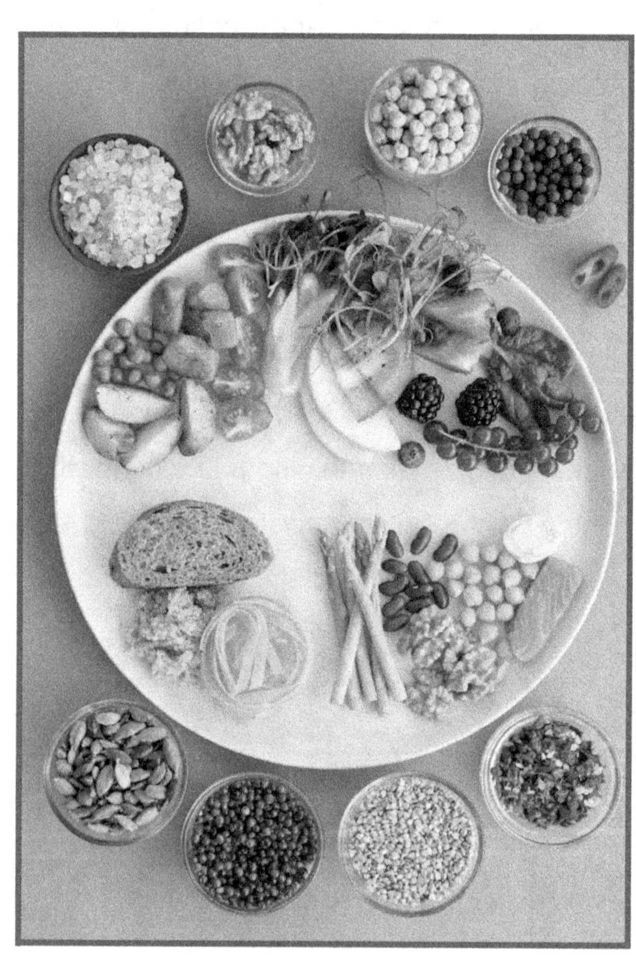

CHAPTER TWO:Causes and Risk Factors

Chronic type 2 diabetes is typified by decreased insulin production and insulin resistance. Several factors contribute to the development of type 2 diabetes, and it often results from a combination of genetic and lifestyle factors. Here's a brief overview of the causes and risk factors:

Genetic Factors

A major contributing factor to the development of type 2 diabetes is genetics. While lifestyle factors such as diet and physical activity contribute to the risk, individuals with a family history of diabetes are more likely to develop the condition. Here are some key points regarding the genetic aspect of type 2 diabetes:

Family History: Having a first-degree relative, such as a parent or sibling, with type 2 diabetes increases an individual's risk. If the illness affects both parents, the risk increases.

Genetic Predisposition: Certain genetic variations and mutations have been associated with an increased susceptibility to type 2 diabetes. These genetic factors can affect insulin production, insulin sensitivity, and other mechanisms involved in glucose metabolism.

Polygenic Inheritance: Type 2 diabetes is considered a polygenic disorder, meaning that multiple genes contribute to its development. The interplay of various genetic factors, along with environmental influences, determines an individual's overall risk.

Heritability: Studies have estimated the heritability of type 2 diabetes to be around

40-70%, indicating a substantial genetic component. However, it's crucial to recognize that genetic predisposition alone is not sufficient to cause diabetes; environmental factors also play a crucial role.

Monogenic Forms: While most cases of type 2 diabetes involve complex interactions between multiple genes and environmental factors, some rare forms result from a single gene mutation. These monogenic forms often present in early adulthood and can be mistaken for type 1 diabetes.

Epigenetics: Beyond genetic variations, epigenetic factors can influence gene expression without altering the underlying DNA sequence. Environmental factors such as diet, stress, and exposure to certain chemicals can modify epigenetic marks, potentially impacting the risk of type 2 diabetes.

Understanding the genetic component of type 2 diabetes can help identify individuals at higher risk and facilitate early interventions. However, genetics is just one piece of the puzzle, and lifestyle factors remain crucial in the prevention and management of the condition. Even individuals with a genetic predisposition can significantly reduce their risk through healthy lifestyle choices, including maintaining a balanced diet, engaging in regular physical activity, and managing weight. Regular medical check-ups and monitoring are important, especially for those with a family history of diabetes.

Lifestyle and Environmental Factors

Lifestyle and environmental factors play a pivotal role in the development of type 2 diabetes. These factors are often modifiable, making them key targets for preventive strategies. Here's an overview:

Obesity and Body Weight: One of the strongest modifiable risk factors for type 2 diabetes is obesity. Excess body fat, especially around the abdomen (visceral fat), is associated with insulin resistance. Preventing diabetes requires maintaining a healthy weight with a balanced diet and regular exercise.

Physical Inactivity: Lack of regular exercise is linked to an increased risk of type 2 diabetes. Physical activity helps improve insulin sensitivity, manage weight, and regulate blood sugar levels. Incorporating regular exercise into one's routine can be an effective strategy for preventing and managing type 2 diabetes.

Dietary Habits: Unhealthy eating patterns, such as a diet high in refined carbohydrates, sugars, and saturated fats, contribute to the development of type 2 diabetes. A diet rich in fruits, vegetables, whole grains, and lean proteins can help control blood sugar levels and reduce the risk of diabetes.

Poor Nutrition and Overconsumption: Consuming an excess of calorie-dense, nutrient-poor foods can lead to weight gain and insulin resistance. Overeating, especially high-calorie snacks and sugary beverages, is associated with an increased risk of type 2 diabetes.

Gestational Diabetes: Women who experience gestational diabetes during pregnancy are at an elevated risk of developing type 2 diabetes later in life. This underscores the importance of monitoring and managing gestational diabetes and maintaining a healthy lifestyle post-pregnancy.

Age: While age itself is a non-modifiable factor, the lifestyle choices made over time contribute to the risk of developing type 2 diabetes. As people age, their metabolism may slow down, and they may become less physically active.

Socioeconomic Factors: Socioeconomic factors, including income, education, and access to healthcare, can influence lifestyle choices. Individuals with lower socioeconomic status may face challenges in accessing nutritious foods, healthcare resources, and opportunities for physical activity.

Stress: Chronic stress can contribute to the development of type 2 diabetes. Stress hormones, such as cortisol, can impact insulin sensitivity. Adopting stress management techniques, such as meditation or exercise, may help mitigate this risk.

Environmental Toxins: Exposure to certain environmental toxins, such as endocrine-disrupting chemicals, has been linked to an increased risk of type 2 diabetes.

These substances can interfere with hormonal regulation and metabolic processes.

Addressing lifestyle and environmental factors through healthy choices and preventive measures is crucial for reducing the risk of type 2 diabetes. Public health initiatives, education, and community interventions play essential roles in promoting healthier lifestyles and creating environments that support diabetes prevention.

Role of Insulin Resistance

A major contributing factor to the onset of type 2 diabetes is insulin resistance. It refers to a condition where the body's cells become less responsive to the effects of insulin, a hormone produced by the pancreas.Because it makes glucose easier for cells to absorb, insulin is essential for controlling blood sugar, or glucose, levels. When cells become resistant to insulin, glucose accumulates in the bloodstream, leading to elevated blood sugar levels. Here's a closer look at the role of insulin resistance in type 2 diabetes:

Normal Insulin Function:

Following a meal, the digestive tract converts carbs into glucose, which is then released into the blood.

In response to rising blood sugar levels, the pancreas releases insulin into the bloodstream.

Insulin acts as a "key" that allows cells, particularly muscle, fat, and liver cells, to take up glucose from the blood.

Once inside the cells, glucose is used for energy or stored for later use.

Insulin Resistance:

In individuals with insulin resistance, cells respond less effectively to the insulin signal.

As a result, the pancreas produces more insulin to compensate for the reduced responsiveness of cells.

This compensatory increase in insulin levels is known as hyperinsulinemia.

Compensatory Mechanisms:

Initially, the pancreas can produce enough insulin to overcome the resistance and maintain normal blood sugar levels.

Over time, however, the pancreas may struggle to keep up with the demand for increased insulin production.

Hyperglycemia:

As insulin resistance progresses, cells become less efficient at taking up glucose, and blood sugar levels rise.

The combination of insulin resistance and elevated blood sugar characterizes prediabetes, a stage that often precedes the diagnosis of type 2 diabetes.

Beta Cell Dysfunction:

The insulin-producing beta cells in the pancreas may also undergo dysfunction over time.

Beta cell dysfunction further contributes to insulin deficiency, exacerbating the imbalance between insulin demand and production.

Vicious Cycle

Insulin resistance and beta cell dysfunction create a vicious cycle, with each factor amplifying the effects of the other.

The result is persistent hyperglycemia, a hallmark of type 2 diabetes.

Consequences of Insulin Resistance:

Insulin resistance is associated with other metabolic abnormalities, including dyslipidemia (abnormal blood lipid levels) and hypertension (high blood pressure).

These factors collectively contribute to the increased risk of cardiovascular disease in individuals with type 2 diabetes.

Addressing insulin resistance is a key focus in the prevention and management of type 2 diabetes. Lifestyle interventions, such as maintaining a healthy weight, engaging in regular physical activity, and adopting a balanced diet, can improve insulin sensitivity and help mitigate the progression of the disease. Medications may also be prescribed to enhance insulin action or reduce glucose production in certain cases.

The Connection with Obesity

The connection between type 2 diabetes and obesity is well-established, and obesity is a significant risk factor for the development of type 2 diabetes. The relationship between the two conditions is complex, involving various mechanisms that contribute to insulin resistance and impaired glucose metabolism. Here are key points regarding the connection between type 2 diabetes and obesity:

Insulin Resistance:

Obesity, especially abdominal or visceral obesity, is strongly associated with insulin resistance.

Excess fat, particularly in the abdominal area, releases substances known as adipokines and free fatty acids, which can interfere with insulin signaling and action.

Insulin resistance makes it difficult for cells, such as those in muscle and fat tissue, to respond effectively to insulin, leading to elevated blood sugar levels.

Adipose Tissue Inflammation:

In obese individuals, adipose (fat) tissue can become inflamed, producing inflammatory cytokines.

Chronic low-grade inflammation is associated with insulin resistance and contributes to the development of type 2 diabetes.

Dyslipidemia:

Obesity is often accompanied by dyslipidemia, characterized by elevated levels of triglycerides and low levels of high-density lipoprotein (HDL or "good" cholesterol).

Dyslipidemia is a metabolic abnormality that can further contribute to insulin resistance.

Adipokines and Hormones:

Adipose tissue secretes various hormones and signaling molecules, collectively known as adipokines.

Some adipokines, such as leptin and adiponectin, play roles in energy balance and insulin sensitivity.

Dysregulation of these adipokines in obesity can contribute to insulin resistance.

Pancreatic Beta Cell Stress:

The increased demand for insulin in obesity can put stress on the insulin-producing beta cells in the pancreas.

Over time, beta cell function may decline, leading to insufficient insulin production and the development of type 2 diabetes.

Inflammatory Pathways:

Obesity is associated with systemic inflammation, and inflammatory pathways can interfere with insulin signaling.

Inflammation may contribute to the progression from insulin resistance to type 2 diabetes.

Weight Loss and Improved Insulin Sensitivity:

Weight loss, achieved through lifestyle changes such as diet and exercise, has been shown to improve insulin sensitivity and reduce the risk of type 2 diabetes.

Even a modest reduction in body weight can have significant benefits in terms of metabolic health.

Central Obesity vs. General Obesity:

The distribution of fat, especially central obesity (fat around the abdomen), appears to be particularly important in the development of insulin resistance and type 2 diabetes.

Genetic Factors:

While genetics also contribute to the risk of type 2 diabetes, the rise in obesity rates globally has paralleled the increased incidence of type 2 diabetes, highlighting the impact of environmental factors, including diet and physical activity.

Addressing obesity through lifestyle modifications, including a balanced diet, regular physical activity, and weight management, is crucial for preventing and managing type 2 diabetes. Additionally, healthcare providers may recommend medications or other interventions to improve insulin sensitivity and glucose metabolism in individuals with obesity and diabetes.

CHAPTER THREE: Diagnosis and Monitoring

Seeking guidance from a healthcare professional in order to receive individualized counsel appropriate to your circumstances is imperative. Always consult with your healthcare team for personalized advice based on your health status and specific needs. They can provide guidance on medication adjustments, lifestyle changes, and overall diabetes management.

Symptoms of Type 2 Diabetes

Type 2 diabetes symptoms can vary, and some people may not experience noticeable symptoms in the early stages. It's essential to be aware of potential signs, and if you suspect you may have diabetes, it's crucial to consult with a healthcare professional for proper evaluation and diagnosis. Common symptoms of type 2 diabetes may include:

Increased Thirst and Hunger: Experiencing excessive thirst (polydipsia) and hunger (polyphagia) may be signs of elevated blood sugar levels.

Frequent Urination: Increased urination (polyuria) can result from the body's attempt to eliminate excess glucose through urine.

Fatigue: Excessive fatigue or low energy levels are common symptoms. This may be related to the body's inability to effectively use glucose for energy.

Unexplained Weight Loss or Gain: Some people with type 2 diabetes may experience unexplained weight loss, while others may gain weight due to increased hunger and overeating.

Blurred Vision: Elevated blood sugar levels can cause changes in the shape of the lens of the eye, leading to blurred vision.

Slow Wound Healing: Diabetes can affect the body's ability to heal wounds and injuries, and infections may take longer to resolve.

Frequent Infections: Individuals with diabetes may be more susceptible to infections, particularly urinary tract infections and skin infections.

Tingling or Numbness: Some people may experience tingling or numbness, especially in the hands or feet. This can be a symptom of nerve damage associated with diabetes (diabetic neuropathy).

Skin Darkening: A condition known as acanthosis nigricans can cause darkening and thickening of the skin, particularly in areas such as the neck, armpits, or groin. This can be associated with insulin resistance.

It's important to note that these symptoms can be subtle or may not be present at all in the early stages of type 2 diabetes. Regular check-ups and blood tests are essential for early detection and effective management. If you suspect you have diabetes or are experiencing any of these symptoms, it is crucial to consult with a healthcare professional for a proper evaluation and diagnosis. Early diagnosis and intervention can help manage the condition and prevent complications.

Diagnostic Tests

The diagnosis of type 2 diabetes involves a combination of clinical assessment and laboratory tests. Healthcare professionals use various diagnostic tools to determine whether an individual has diabetes, and these tests help in understanding the severity of the condition. Here are some comprehensive diagnostic tests for a type 2 diabetic patient:

Fasting Blood Sugar Test (FBS):

Purpose: Measures blood glucose levels after an overnight fast.

Procedure: The patient fasts for at least 8 hours, and a blood sample is taken to measure fasting blood sugar levels.

Results: A fasting blood sugar level of 126 milligrams per deciliter (mg/dL) or higher on two separate occasions generally indicates diabetes.

Oral Glucose Tolerance Test (OGTT):

Purpose: Assesses how the body handles glucose after consuming a sugary drink.

Procedure: The patient fasts overnight, then drinks a solution containing a specific amount of glucose. Periodically, blood samples are drawn to monitor the body's glucose metabolism.

Results: A 2-hour blood sugar level of 200 mg/dL or higher suggests diabetes.

Hemoglobin A1c Test:

Purpose: Provides an average of blood sugar levels over the past 2-3 months.

Procedure: A blood sample is taken, and the result is presented as a percentage.

Results: An A1c level of 6.5% or higher is indicative of diabetes.

Random Blood Sugar Test:

Purpose: Measures blood sugar levels at any time of the day, without fasting.

Procedure: A blood sample is taken without regard to the time of the last meal.

Results: A blood sugar level of 200 mg/dL or higher, along with symptoms of diabetes, may indicate diabetes.

Glycated Albumin (GA) Test:

Purpose: Measures the percentage of glycated albumin in the blood.

Procedure: A blood sample is taken to assess the level of glycated albumin.

Results: Elevated levels may suggest poor blood sugar control over the past few weeks.

C-peptide Test:

Purpose: Measures the amount of insulin produced by the pancreas.

Procedure: A blood sample is taken to measure C-peptide levels.

Results: Low C-peptide levels may indicate decreased insulin production, which is common in advanced type 2 diabetes.

Insulin Resistance Test:

Purpose: Assesses the body's response to insulin.

Procedure: Various methods, such as the Homeostasis Model Assessment of Insulin Resistance (HOMA-IR), can be used to estimate insulin resistance.

Results: Higher values indicate greater insulin resistance.

Lipid Profile:

Purpose: Assesses lipid levels, including cholesterol and triglycerides.

Procedure: A blood sample is taken to measure lipid levels.

Results: Abnormal lipid levels may be associated with insulin resistance and metabolic syndrome, common in type 2 diabetes.

Diagnosing and monitoring type 2 diabetes require a multidimensional approach, considering various factors and tests. It's crucial for healthcare professionals to interpret results in the context of an individual's overall health and medical history. Regular follow-up tests and monitoring help in adjusting treatment plans and managing the condition effectively.

Blood Sugar Monitoring

Blood sugar monitoring is a critical aspect of managing type 2 diabetes. Regular monitoring helps individuals with diabetes and their healthcare providers understand how well blood sugar levels are being controlled, enabling adjustments to treatment plans as needed. Here's an overview of blood sugar monitoring in type 2 diabetes:

Importance of Blood Sugar Monitoring:

Treatment Adjustment: Regular monitoring provides valuable information to adjust medications, lifestyle, and dietary choices to maintain optimal blood sugar levels.

Prevention of Complications: Consistent blood sugar control helps prevent complications associated with diabetes, such as heart disease, kidney problems, nerve damage, and vision issues.

Individualized Care: Monitoring allows for personalized diabetes management, taking into account the unique needs and responses of each individual.

Methods of Blood Sugar Monitoring:

Glucometers:

Description: Portable devices that measure blood sugar levels using a small drop of blood, usually obtained by pricking the fingertip.

Frequency: Patients may check their blood sugar multiple times a day, especially before meals and bedtime.

Continuous Glucose Monitoring (CGM):

Description: A system that continuously tracks blood sugar levels throughout the day and night via a small sensor inserted under the skin.

Benefits: Provides real-time data, trend information, and alerts for high or low blood sugar levels.

Usage: Suitable for individuals requiring frequent monitoring or those at risk of severe hypoglycemia.

Blood Sugar Targets:

Fasting Blood Sugar:

Target Range: Usually between 80-130 mg/dL before meals.

Postprandial Blood Sugar (After Meals):

Target Range: Typically below 180 mg/dL, measured 1-2 hours after the start of a meal.

Hemoglobin A1c (A1c) Levels:

Target Range: Generally below 7%, although individual targets may vary.

Tips for Effective Blood Sugar Monitoring:

Consistency is Key:

Perform blood sugar checks at consistent times each day to identify patterns and trends.

Record Keeping:

Maintain a log of blood sugar readings, meals, physical activity, and medication doses. This information can assist healthcare providers in making informed decisions.

Understand Your Numbers:

Learn to interpret blood sugar readings and understand the impact of food, exercise, and medications on blood sugar levels.

Communication with Healthcare Team:

Share blood sugar records with healthcare providers during regular check-ups to facilitate collaborative decision-making.

Education:

Stay informed about the latest advancements in blood sugar monitoring technology and techniques to make informed choices about managing diabetes.

Challenges and Considerations:

Variability:

Blood sugar levels can fluctuate due to various factors, including stress, illness, and changes in routine.

Hypoglycemia Awareness:

Individuals on certain medications, especially insulin, need to be vigilant about recognizing and managing low blood sugar levels (hypoglycemia).

Technology Limitations:

While advanced technologies like CGM offer continuous monitoring, they may not be suitable for everyone due to factors like cost and personal preferences.

Blood sugar monitoring is a crucial tool in the comprehensive management of type 2 diabetes. It empowers individuals to make informed decisions about their health, promotes effective communication with healthcare providers, and contributes to long-term well-being. Regular discussions with healthcare teams help ensure that blood sugar targets are personalized and achievable based on individual circumstances.

Importance of Regular Check-ups

Regular check-ups are of paramount importance in the management of type 2 diabetes. These appointments serve as crucial opportunities for healthcare professionals to monitor and assess various aspects of a patient's health, providing valuable insights into the effectiveness of diabetes management strategies. Here's an emphasis on the importance of regular check-ups for individuals with type 2 diabetes:

1. Early Detection and Diagnosis:

Regular check-ups allow for the early detection and diagnosis of complications associated with diabetes, such as cardiovascular disease, kidney problems, and eye issues. Early intervention can prevent or mitigate the impact of these complications.

2. Blood Sugar Monitoring and Adjustment:

Healthcare professionals use regular check-ups to review blood sugar monitoring records. By analyzing trends and patterns, they can make necessary adjustments to medication regimens, insulin doses, or other treatment plans to optimize blood sugar control.

3. Medication Management:

Check-ups provide opportunities to assess the effectiveness of prescribed medications and make any necessary adjustments. This ensures that patients are on the most suitable medications to manage their diabetes and associated conditions.

4. Comprehensive Health Assessment:

Beyond blood sugar control, regular check-ups include a comprehensive assessment of overall health. This may involve checking blood pressure, cholesterol levels, kidney function, and other relevant health markers.

5. Lifestyle Counseling:

Healthcare providers use check-ups to offer guidance on lifestyle factors, such as diet, exercise, and stress management. These discussions help individuals with type 2 diabetes make informed choices that contribute to overall well-being.

6. Preventive Measures:

Regular check-ups enable healthcare professionals to identify potential risk factors for complications and implement preventive measures. This proactive approach can significantly reduce the likelihood of developing serious health issues.

7. Educational Opportunities:

Check-ups provide opportunities for healthcare providers to educate individuals with type 2 diabetes about the latest developments in diabetes management, lifestyle modifications, and self-care practices. Education empowers patients to actively participate in their own health management.

8. Emotional Well-being:

Living with a chronic condition like diabetes can impact mental and emotional well-being. Regular check-ups provide a platform for individuals to discuss any emotional challenges they may be facing, and healthcare professionals can offer support and resources.

9. Review of Self-Monitoring:

If individuals are using tools like blood glucose meters or continuous glucose monitors for self-monitoring, regular check-ups allow healthcare providers to review this data. This can lead to insights into daily patterns, adherence to monitoring regimens, and adjustments to improve outcomes.

10. Individualized Care Plans:

Regular check-ups facilitate the development of individualized care plans based on each patient's unique needs, preferences, and responses to treatment. This personalized approach enhances the effectiveness of diabetes management.

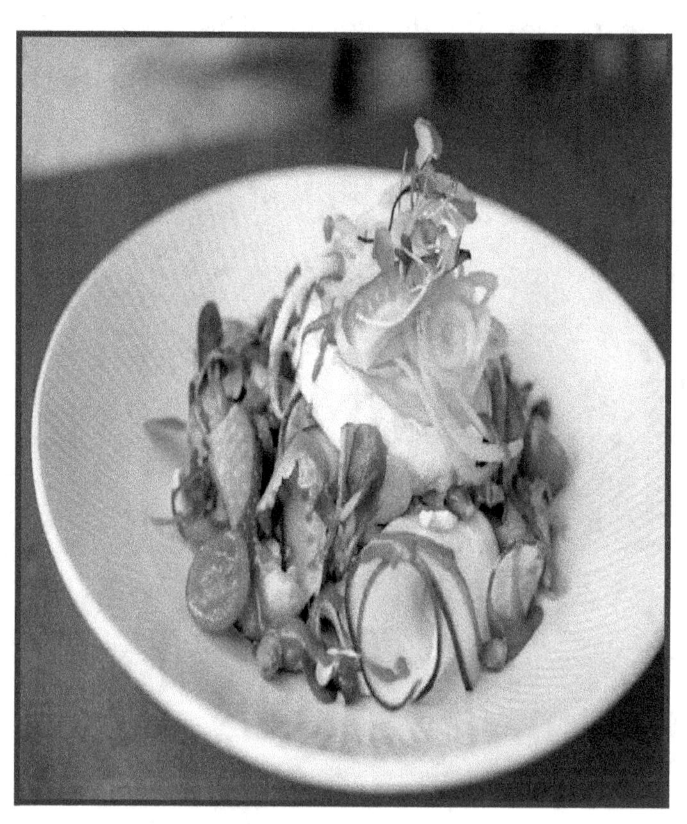

f

CHAPTER FOUR: Lifestyle Changes for Diabetes Management

The Role of Diet in Managing Type 2 Diabetes

Managing type 2 diabetes involves a combination of lifestyle changes, and diet plays a crucial role in maintaining blood sugar levels. Here's an overview of the role of diet in managing type 2 diabetes:

Understanding Carbohydrates

Carbohydrates have the most significant impact on blood sugar levels. They are broken down into glucose, raising blood sugar levels. Therefore, it's important to monitor and manage carbohydrate intake.

Focus on complex carbohydrates like whole grains, legumes, and vegetables, which have a slower impact on blood sugar compared to simple carbohydrates found in processed foods.

Portion Control:

Controlling portion sizes helps regulate calorie intake and blood sugar levels. Eating smaller, balanced meals throughout the day can prevent spikes in blood sugar.

Use smaller plates to visually control portions, and be mindful of portion sizes when eating out.

Choose Healthy Fats:

Opt for heart-healthy fats such as avocados, nuts, seeds, and olive oil. These fats have a minimal impact on blood sugar and provide essential nutrients.

Reduce your intake of processed snacks, fried foods, and some oils that contain saturated and trans fats.

Include Lean Proteins:

Protein keeps you feeling full and helps to normalize blood sugar levels. Pick lean protein sources such as beans, lentils, fish, poultry, and tofu.

Avoid processed meats and opt for healthier cooking methods like grilling, baking, or steaming.

Fiber-Rich Foods:

Fiber helps to control blood sugar levels by slowing down the absorption of sugar. Make sure your diet is rich in whole grains, legumes, fruits, and veggies.

Try to consume 25–30 grams of fiber per day, minimum.

Limit Added Sugars:

Minimize the intake of foods and beverages with added sugars. Check food labels for hidden sugars like high-fructose corn syrup, sucrose, or other sweeteners.

Opt for natural sweeteners like stevia or moderate amounts of honey or maple syrup.
Regular Meal Timing:

Establish a regular eating schedule with consistent meal times. Spreading meals throughout the day can help prevent large spikes or drops in blood sugar levels.
Snack on healthy options like nuts, yogurt, or vegetables between meals if needed.

Stay Hydrated:
Adequate hydration is important for overall health. Choose water or other sugar-free beverages to stay hydrated.
Limit sugary drinks like sodas and fruit juices.Check-ups are the cornerstone of effective type 2 diabetes management. They offer a holistic approach to care, addressing not only blood sugar control but also various aspects of overall health and well-being. Consistent follow-up with healthcare providers

helps individuals navigate the complexities of diabetes, minimize complications, and lead healthier lives. It is crucial for individuals with type 2 diabetes to actively engage in and prioritize regular check-ups as an integral part of their healthcare routine.

Carbohydrates, Proteins, and Fats

Managing carbohydrates, proteins, and fats is crucial for individuals with type 2 diabetes to maintain stable blood sugar levels and overall health. Here's an overview of each macronutrient in the context of type 2 diabetes:

1. Carbohydrates:

Role in the Diet:

The body uses carbohydrates as its main energy source.They are broken down into glucose, which is used by cells for fuel.

Managing carbohydrate intake is critical for people with type 2 diabetes as it directly affects blood sugar levels.

Types of Carbohydrates:

Complex Carbohydrates: Found in whole grains, vegetables, legumes, and fruits. They have a slower impact on blood sugar due to their fiber content, which helps regulate glucose absorption.

Simple Carbohydrates: Found in sugars and processed foods. They can cause rapid spikes in blood sugar levels and should be limited.

Dietary Tips:

Focus on whole, unprocessed foods with high fiber content.

Select whole grains over refined grains, such as quinoa, brown rice, and whole wheat.

Be mindful of portion sizes and distribute carbohydrate intake throughout the day.

2. Proteins:

Role in the Diet:

Proteins are essential for building and repairing tissues, and they contribute to a feeling of fullness.

Including lean protein sources in the diet can help stabilize blood sugar levels.

Types of Proteins:

Lean Proteins: Found in poultry, fish, tofu, legumes, and lean cuts of meat. These sources are lower in saturated fats.

Fatty Proteins: Found in processed meats and certain cuts of red meat. Consumption of these should be limited.

Dietary Tips:

Include a variety of lean protein sources in your diet.

Limit processed meats and opt for healthier cooking methods like grilling, baking, or steaming.

3. Fats:

Role in the Diet:

Fats are essential for absorbing fat-soluble vitamins (A, D, E, and K) and are a concentrated source of energy.

Choosing healthy fats is crucial for cardiovascular health, especially for individuals with type 2 diabetes who may be at a higher risk of heart disease.

Types of Fats:

Healthy Fats: Nuts, seeds, avocados, olive oil, and fatty seafood are good sources of healthy fats. These fats are heart-healthy and can help manage cholesterol levels.

Unhealthy Fats: Found in trans fats and saturated fats present in fried foods, processed snacks, and certain oils. These should be limited.

Dietary Tips:

Prioritize sources of healthy fats in your diet.

Limit the intake of saturated and trans fats to reduce the risk of cardiovascular complications.

General Dietary Tips for Type 2 Diabetes:

Balanced Meals: Make sure that every meal consists of a mix of fats, proteins, and carbohydrates.

Portion Control: To control calorie consumption, pay attention to portion sizes.

Fiber-Rich Foods: Include plenty of fruits, vegetables, and whole grains for added fiber.

Regular Meal Timing: Establish consistent meal times to help regulate blood sugar levels.

Hydration: Drink water or other sugar-free beverages to stay hydrated.

Consult Healthcare Professionals: Work with your healthcare team to create a personalized meal plan based on your specific needs.

Always consult with healthcare professionals, including a registered dietitian or nutritionist, to tailor dietary recommendations to your individual health condition and medication requirements.

Glycemic Index and Load

Understanding the concepts of Glycemic Index (GI) and Glycemic Load (GL) can be beneficial for managing blood sugar levels in individuals with type 2 diabetes.

1. Glycemic Index (GI):

Definition: The Glycemic Index is a scale that ranks carbohydrates in foods based on how quickly they raise blood sugar levels.

Scale: Foods are assigned a value on a scale from 0 to 100, with higher values indicating a faster and larger increase in blood sugar levels.

Categories:

Low GI (55 or less): Foods that cause a slower and lower rise in blood sugar.

Medium GI (56-69): Foods that cause a moderate rise in blood sugar.

High GI (70 and above): Foods that cause a rapid and higher rise in blood sugar.

Implications for Type 2 Diabetes:

Choosing low-GI foods can help manage blood sugar levels more effectively.

Low-GI foods tend to provide a more sustained release of glucose, leading to better blood sugar control.

Examples of low-GI foods include most fruits and vegetables, whole grains, and legumes.

2. Glycemic Load (GL):

Definition: Glycemic Load takes into account both the quality (GI) and quantity of carbohydrates in a particular serving of food.

Calculation: GL is calculated by multiplying the GI of a food by the amount of carbohydrates it contains and dividing by 100.

Categories:

Low GL (10 or less): Foods that have a minimal impact on blood sugar.

Medium GL (11-19): Foods with a moderate impact on blood sugar.

High GL (20 and above): Foods that can cause a significant rise in blood sugar.

Implications for Type 2 Diabetes:

Considering both GI and GL provides a more comprehensive understanding of how a specific food affects blood sugar levels.

Lowering overall glycemic load can be beneficial for managing blood sugar levels in individuals with type 2 diabetes.

Choosing a combination of low-GI and moderate-GL foods can contribute to better blood sugar control.

Practical Tips for Type 2 Diabetes Management:

Choose Whole, Unprocessed Foods: Whole grains, fruits, vegetables, and legumes often have lower GIs and contribute to a lower GL.

Combine Foods: Combining low-GI foods with proteins and healthy fats can further reduce the overall impact on blood sugar.

Monitor Portion Sizes: Controlling portion sizes helps manage the total glycemic load of a meal.

Be Mindful of Cooking Methods: Some cooking methods, like boiling or steaming, can help maintain the low-GI nature of certain foods.

Include Fiber: Foods high in fiber tend to have lower GIs and can help slow down the absorption of glucose.

Individualized Approach: Keep in mind that individual responses to foods can vary. One person's solution might not be another's.

Consult Healthcare Professionals: Work with healthcare providers, including dietitians or nutritionists, to develop a personalized dietary plan based on individual health conditions and needs.

Understanding the concepts of GI and GL and incorporating this knowledge into dietary choices can be a valuable tool for managing blood sugar levels in individuals with type 2 diabetes. However, it's crucial to consider these factors alongside an overall balanced and individualized approach to diet and lifestyle.Seek individual counsel from healthcare professionals at all times.

Portion Control

Portion control is a crucial aspect of managing type 2 diabetes because it helps regulate calorie intake, maintain a healthy weight, and control blood sugar levels. Here are some key considerations for portion control in individuals with type 2 diabetes:

1. Understanding Portion Sizes:

Many people underestimate portion sizes, leading to excess calorie intake. Acquire the ability to identify suitable serving sizes for various food categories.

2. Balanced Meals:

Aim for well-balanced meals that include a mix of carbohydrates, proteins, and healthy fats. This helps provide sustained energy and prevents large fluctuations in blood sugar levels.

3. Use Smaller Plates and Bowls:

Using smaller plates and bowls can create an optical illusion, making portions appear larger. This psychological trick may help control the amount of food consumed.

4. Half-Plate Rule:

Divide your plate into half. Fill half with non-starchy vegetables, one-quarter with lean protein, and one-quarter with whole grains or starchy vegetables. This visually helps control portion sizes.

5. Read Food Labels:

Pay attention to serving sizes on food labels. Nutritional information is often presented per serving, and it's important to be aware of what constitutes a single serving.

6. Mindful Eating:

Eat slowly and savor each bite. Recognize your signs of hunger and fullness to prevent overindulging. Being mindful allows better control over portion sizes.

7. Avoid Second Helpings:

Resist the temptation to go for second helpings. Wait for a few minutes after finishing your first serving to assess whether you are still hungry.

8. Limit Liquid Calories:

Be mindful of liquid calories, including sugary drinks and alcohol. These can contribute to excess calorie intake without providing a feeling of fullness.

9. Snack Smartly:

Choose healthy snacks and portion them out in advance. Pre-portioning snacks helps avoid mindless eating.

10. Plan Meals in Advance:

Plan your meals and snacks ahead of time. This helps you make intentional choices about portion sizes and avoid impulsive decisions.

11. Restaurant Awareness:

When dining out, consider sharing a dish or asking for a smaller portion. Restaurant servings are often larger than necessary.

12. Weighing and Measuring:

Initially, measuring and weighing food can provide a better understanding of portion sizes. Over time, this knowledge becomes intuitive.

13. Consult with a Dietitian:

Work with a registered dietitian or nutritionist to create a personalized meal plan that aligns with your specific dietary needs, considering factors like age, activity level, and medications.

14. Regular Monitoring:

Regularly monitor blood sugar levels to understand how different portions and food choices impact your body.

15. Physical Activity:

Incorporate regular physical activity into your routine. Exercise can help with weight management and improve insulin sensitivity.

Remember that individual nutritional needs vary, and it's important to tailor portion control strategies to your specific health conditions and preferences. Adopting a sustainable, balanced approach to portion control can contribute significantly to the effective management of type 2 diabetes.

Importance of Regular Exercise

Regular exercise is a cornerstone in the management and prevention of type 2 diabetes. It offers a multitude of benefits that contribute to better blood sugar control, improved insulin sensitivity, and overall health. Here's an overview of the importance of regular exercise in type 2 diabetes:

1. Enhanced Insulin Sensitivity:

Exercise helps the body use insulin more efficiently. This increased sensitivity allows cells to take up and use glucose more effectively, resulting in better blood sugar control.

2. Blood Sugar Regulation:

Physical activity helps regulate blood sugar levels by promoting the movement of glucose from the bloodstream into cells, where it is used for energy. This can lead to lower fasting and post-meal blood sugar levels.

3. Weight Management:

Regular exercise plays a crucial role in weight management, which is essential for individuals with type 2 diabetes. Maintaining a healthy weight can improve insulin sensitivity and reduce the risk of complications.

4. Cardiovascular Health:

Type 2 diabetes is often associated with an increased risk of cardiovascular disease. Exercise strengthens the cardiovascular system, improving heart health and reducing the risk of heart-related complications.

5. Improved Lipid Profile:

Physical activity can positively impact lipid profiles by increasing high-density lipoprotein (HDL or "good" cholesterol) and decreasing triglycerides. Better overall cardiovascular health is a result of this.

6. Muscle Glucose Uptake:

Working muscles during exercise take up glucose without the need for insulin, providing an alternative way to manage blood sugar levels.

7. Stress Reduction:

It is commonly recognized that exercise lowers stress and enhances mental health. Stress management is important for people with diabetes, as stress hormones can affect blood sugar levels.

8. Enhanced Weight Loss and Maintenance:

Exercise, combined with a healthy diet, supports weight loss and helps individuals maintain a healthy weight. This is crucial for managing type 2 diabetes and reducing the risk of obesity-related complications.

9. Prevention of Complications:

Regular physical activity can help prevent or delay the onset of diabetes-related complications, such as cardiovascular disease, nerve damage, and kidney problems.

10. Improved Sleep Patterns:

Exercise can contribute to better sleep quality. Poor sleep patterns have been linked to insulin resistance and an increased risk of type 2 diabetes.

11. Types of Exercise:

Aerobic exercises (e.g., walking, jogging, cycling) and resistance training (e.g., weightlifting) both offer benefits for individuals with type 2 diabetes. A combination of both is often recommended.

12. Consistency is Key:

Regularity in exercise is crucial for sustained benefits. Consistent physical activity helps maintain the positive effects on blood sugar control and overall health.

13. Consultation with Healthcare Professionals:

Before starting an exercise program, individuals with type 2 diabetes should consult with their healthcare team to ensure that the chosen activities align with their health condition and medication regimen.

14. Personalized Approach:

Exercise plans should be tailored to individual abilities, preferences, and health status. This ensures a sustainable and enjoyable routine.

Regular exercise is a powerful tool in the management of type 2 diabetes. It not only helps control blood sugar levels but also contributes to overall health and well-being. Individuals with diabetes are encouraged to incorporate physical activity into their daily routine and work closely with healthcare professionals to develop a safe and effective exercise plan.

Exercise

For individuals with type 2 diabetes, a well-rounded exercise routine should include a combination of aerobic exercises, strength training, flexibility exercises, and balance training. Here's a breakdown of each type of exercise and why they are beneficial for managing type 2 diabetes:

1. Aerobic Exercises:

Definition: These are activities that increase your heart rate and breathing. They improve cardiovascular health and help control blood sugar levels.

Examples:

Brisk walking

Jogging or running

Cycling

Swimming

Dancing

Aerobics classes

Benefits:

Improves insulin sensitivity.

Helps lower blood sugar levels.

Aids in weight management.

Enhances cardiovascular health.

2. Strength Training:

Definition: Involves using resistance to build and tone muscles. It's important for preserving muscle mass, improving metabolism, and aiding in blood sugar control.

Examples:

Weightlifting

Bodyweight exercises (e.g., squats, lunges, push-ups)

Resistance band exercises

Benefits:

Enhances insulin sensitivity.

Supports weight management.

Preserves and builds muscle mass.

Boosts metabolism.

3. Flexibility Exercises:

Definition: Stretching activities that improve flexibility and range of motion. While not directly impacting blood sugar, they are crucial for overall well-being and injury prevention.

Examples:

Yoga

Pilates

Stretching exercises

Benefits:

Improves flexibility and joint health.

Reduces the risk of injuries.

Enhances overall physical function.

4. Balance Training:

Definition: Exercises that improve balance and stability. Important for preventing falls, especially for older individuals with diabetes who may have neuropathy.

Examples:

Tai Chi

Balance exercises on one leg

Stability ball exercises

Benefits:

Reduces the risk of falls and injuries.

Enhances overall stability.

5. Interval Training:

Definition: Alternating between short bursts of intense activity and periods of rest or lower-intensity exercise. Can be applied to both aerobic and strength exercises.

Examples:

High-Intensity Interval Training (HIIT)

Interval walking or jogging

Benefits:

Improves cardiovascular fitness.

Can be time-efficient.

Enhances insulin sensitivity.

6. Walking:

Definition: Walking is a low-impact aerobic exercise that is accessible and can be easily incorporated into daily life.

Benefits:

Improves cardiovascular health.

Aids in weight management.

Regulates blood sugar levels.

General Tips:

Consult with Healthcare Professionals:

Before starting any exercise program, consult with your healthcare team to ensure that your chosen activities align with your health condition and medications.

Gradual Progression:

To avoid injuries, start out carefully and increase the duration and intensity of your workouts gradually.

Regular Monitoring:

Monitor your blood sugar levels regularly, especially before and after exercise, to understand how different activities affect you.

Stay Hydrated:

Drink plenty of water before, during, and after exercise to stay hydrated.

Consistency is Key:

Aim for regular, consistent exercise to reap the long-term benefits.

Remember that individual preferences, fitness levels, and health conditions vary. A combination of these exercises, tailored to your preferences and physical condition, can contribute significantly to the management of type 2 diabetes. Always seek guidance from healthcare professionals or fitness experts to create a personalized exercise plan.

Strength Training

Strength training, also known as resistance training or weightlifting, is an important component of type 2 diabetes management. While aerobic exercise is commonly emphasized, incorporating strength training into your fitness routine offers specific benefits for individuals with type 2 diabetes. Here's why strength training is valuable and how it can contribute to diabetes management:

1. Improved Insulin Sensitivity:

Strength training has been shown to enhance insulin sensitivity, allowing the body to use insulin more effectively.Over time, this may result in improved blood sugar regulation.

2. Glucose Metabolism:

Resistance training can improve glucose metabolism by increasing the uptake of glucose by muscle cells, independent of insulin. This is particularly beneficial for individuals with insulin resistance, a common feature of type 2 diabetes.

3. Blood Sugar Regulation:

Regular strength training can help regulate blood sugar levels by utilizing glucose for energy during and after exercise. This effect persists even after the workout is completed.

4. Muscle Mass Preservation:

Type 2 diabetes is associated with a risk of muscle loss. Strength training helps preserve and build lean muscle mass, which is important for metabolic health, weight management, and functional ability.

5. Weight Management:

Building muscle through strength training contributes to an increase in basal metabolic rate (BMR), aiding in weight management. Maintaining a healthy weight is crucial for individuals with type 2 diabetes.

6. Improved Cardiovascular Health:

While aerobic exercise is known for cardiovascular benefits, strength training also has positive effects. It can lead to improvements in blood pressure and lipid profiles, reducing the risk of heart-related complications associated with diabetes.

7. Enhanced Physical Function:

Strength training improves overall physical function, making daily activities easier to perform. This can have a positive impact on quality of life, especially for older adults with diabetes.

8. Joint Health and Bone Density:

Resistance training supports joint health and can help maintain or increase bone density. This is particularly important for individuals with diabetes, as they may be at a higher risk of bone-related issues.

9. Individualized Approach:

Strength training programs can be tailored to individual fitness levels and health conditions. This makes it accessible and beneficial for people of various ages and abilities.

10. Combination with Aerobic Exercise:

Combining strength training with aerobic exercise creates a comprehensive fitness routine. Both types of exercise offer unique benefits for diabetes management.

11. Consistency and Gradual Progression:

Consistency is key in strength training. Starting with a manageable intensity and gradually progressing ensures safety and sustainability.

12. Consultation with Healthcare Professionals:

Individuals with type 2 diabetes should consult with their healthcare team before starting a strength training program. This ensures that the chosen activities align with their health status and any existing complications.

13. Varied Exercises:

A well-rounded strength training routine includes exercises targeting different muscle groups. This can involve using machines, resistance bands, free weights, or bodyweight workouts.

Incorporating strength training into a diabetes management plan offers a holistic approach to health and well-being. It complements other lifestyle modifications such as dietary changes and aerobic exercise, contributing to overall glycemic control and reducing the risk of complications associated with type 2 diabetes. Always seek guidance from healthcare professionals or fitness experts to develop a safe and effective strength training program tailored to individual needs.

Flexibility and Balance Exercises

For individuals living with type 2 diabetes, incorporating flexibility and balance exercises into your routine is important for overall health and well-being. Here's why these types of exercises are beneficial and some examples you might consider:

1. Flexibility Exercises:

Flexibility exercises focus on improving the range of motion of your joints and muscles. They enhance your ability to move easily and can contribute to better overall physical function.

Benefits:

Joint Health: Improves the flexibility of joints, reducing stiffness and the risk of injury.

Posture: Enhances posture and alignment, reducing the likelihood of musculoskeletal issues.

Mobility: Increases the range of motion, making daily activities more manageable.

Examples:

Yoga: Combines stretching, strength, and balancing exercises with breath control.

Pilates: Emphasizes core strength, flexibility, and overall body awareness.

Static Stretching: Holding a stretch position for a set period to lengthen muscles.

2. Balance Exercises:

Exercises for balance are meant to increase stability and lower the chance of falling. They become especially important for individuals with diabetes, who may be at a higher risk of neuropathy (nerve damage).

Benefits:

Fall Prevention: Improves balance, reducing the risk of falls, which can be crucial for those with diabetes-related neuropathy.

Functional Ability: Enhances overall stability, making daily activities safer and more manageable.

Joint and Muscle Control: Strengthens the muscles that support joints, improving overall joint control.

Examples:

Tai Chi: A low-impact exercise that combines slow, flowing movements with deep breathing and meditation.

One-Leg Stands: Stand on one leg for a short duration, gradually increasing the time as your balance improves.

Heel-to-Toe Walking: Maintain a straight gait while putting one foot's heel in front of the other's toes.

Incorporating Flexibility and Balance Exercises:

Consistency: Aim for at least two to three sessions per week for flexibility exercises and daily practice for balance exercises.

Warm-up: Always start with a gentle warm-up before engaging in flexibility exercises to prepare your muscles.

Listen to Your Body: Pay attention to how your body feels during exercises. If you experience pain or discomfort, modify the exercise or stop and consult your healthcare team.

Progress Gradually: Whether you are new to these exercises or returning after a break, progress gradually to prevent injuries.

Enjoy Variety: Keep your routine interesting by trying different flexibility and balance exercises to target various muscle groups.

Precautions for Individuals with Diabetes:

Foot Care: Check your feet regularly for any cuts, sores, or blisters, especially if you have neuropathy.

Hydration: Stay well-hydrated, particularly if you're engaging in activities that make you sweat.

Blood Sugar Monitoring: Monitor your blood sugar levels before and after exercise to understand its impact on your levels.

Footwear: Wear proper footwear with good support and traction to reduce the risk of slipping.

Remember to consult with your healthcare team before starting any new exercise program, especially if you have pre-existing health conditions or concerns. They can provide personalized advice based on your individual health status and help you create a safe and effective flexibility and balance exercise routine.

Stress Management Techniques

Stress management is an essential aspect of managing type 2 diabetes. Chronic stress can impact blood sugar levels and overall health. Adopting effective stress management techniques can contribute to better glycemic control and improve the overall well-being of individuals with diabetes. The following stress-reduction methods could be useful

1. Mindfulness Meditation:

Description: Mindfulness involves staying present and fully engaging in the current moment. Meditation techniques, such as focused breathing or body scan meditations, can help reduce stress and promote relaxation.

Benefits:

Lowers stress hormone levels.

Improves emotional well-being.

Enhances overall mental clarity.

2. Deep Breathing Exercises:

Description: Deep breathing exercises, such as diaphragmatic breathing or box breathing, can activate the body's relaxation response, reducing stress.

Benefits:

Calms the nervous system.

Promotes relaxation.

Improves focus and concentration.

3. Progressive Muscle Relaxation (PMR):

Description: PMR involves systematically tensing and then relaxing different muscle groups, promoting physical and mental relaxation.

Benefits:

Reduces muscle tension.

Enhances overall relaxation.

Can be easily practiced anywhere.

4. Yoga:

Description: Yoga combines physical postures, breath control, and meditation. It is highly renowned for its capacity to lower stress and enhance general wellbeing.

Benefits:

Improves flexibility and strength.

Reduces stress and anxiety.

Enhances mindfulness.

5. Guided Imagery:

Description: Guided imagery involves visualizing calming and peaceful scenes, helping to shift focus away from stressors.

Benefits:

Reduces stress and anxiety.

Promotes a sense of calm.

Enhances mental well-being.

6. Regular Physical Activity:

Description: Engaging in regular exercise, such as walking, jogging, or other forms of physical activity, can be an effective way to manage stress.

Benefits:

Releases endorphins, which improve mood.

Reduces stress hormones.

Enhances overall physical and mental health.

7. Social Support:

Description: Sharing your feelings and concerns with friends, family, or support groups can provide emotional support and help manage stress.

Benefits:

Provides a sense of connection.

Offers emotional support.

Encourages problem-solving.

8. Time Management:

Description: Effectively managing time and setting priorities can reduce the feeling of being overwhelmed and stressed.

Benefits:

Improves efficiency.

Reduces stress related to deadlines.

Enhances a sense of control.

9. Cognitive Behavioral Therapy (CBT):

Description: CBT is a therapeutic approach that helps individuals identify and change negative thought patterns and behaviors contributing to stress.

Benefits:

Promotes positive thinking.

Improves coping strategies.

Reduces anxiety and stress.

10. Hobbies and Leisure Activities:

Description: Engaging in activities you enjoy, such as reading, gardening, or artistic pursuits, can provide a healthy distraction from stressors.

Benefits:

Fosters a sense of enjoyment.

Offers a break from daily stress.

Promotes a positive mindset.

Integrating stress management techniques into your daily life is an important part of managing type 2 diabetes. Experiment with different approaches to find what works best for you, and consider incorporating these techniques into your routine to support both your mental and physical health.

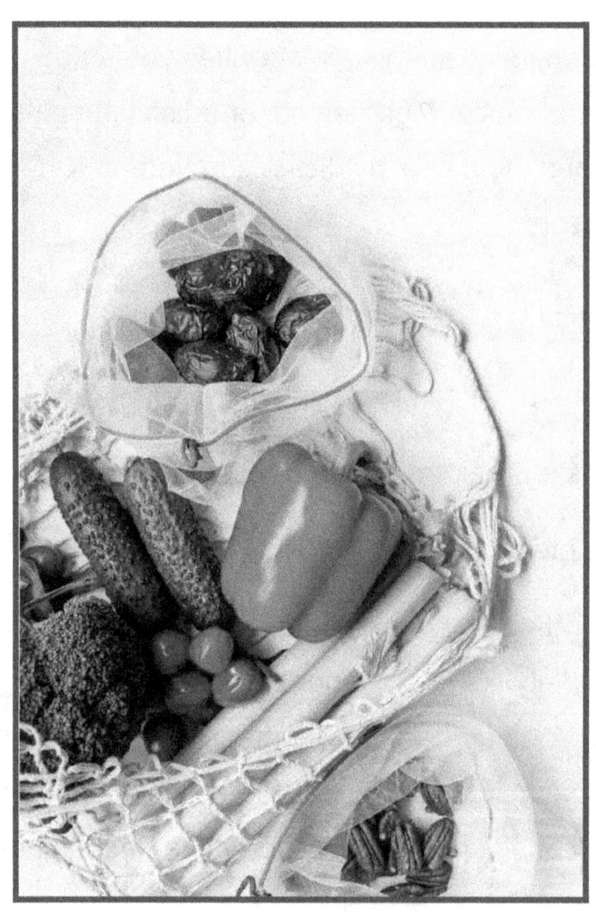

CHAPTER FIVE: Nutrition Essentials

Foods to Include in Your Diet: Diabetes-Friendly Superfoods

If you have diabetes, maintaining a healthy and balanced diet is crucial for managing blood sugar levels and overall well-being. Including diabetes-friendly superfoods in your diet can offer nutritional benefits and help control blood sugar. Here are some superfoods to consider:

Berries:

Antioxidants, fiber, and vitamins abound in berries including raspberries, strawberries, and blueberries. They have a low glycemic index, which means they have a smaller impact on blood sugar levels.

Fatty Fish:

Omega-3 fatty acids are abundant in fatty fish, such as sardines, mackerel, and salmon. These fats may reduce inflammation, improve heart health, and help manage insulin resistance.

Leafy Greens:

Dark, leafy greens such as spinach, kale, and Swiss chard are packed with nutrients like vitamins, minerals, and antioxidants. They are also low in carbohydrates, making them a good choice for diabetes management.

Nuts and Seeds:

Good fats, fiber, and protein can be found in plenty in almonds, walnuts, chia seeds, flaxseeds, and pumpkin seeds. They can be a satisfying and blood sugar-friendly snack.

Whole Grains:

Opt for whole grains like quinoa, barley, brown rice, and oats over refined grains. Whole grains provide fiber, which helps regulate blood sugar levels and contributes to overall digestive health.

Greek Yogurt:

Greek yogurt is a good source of protein and probiotics. Choose plain, unsweetened varieties to avoid added sugars. The protein content can help with satiety and blood sugar control.

Cinnamon:

The ability of cinnamon to increase insulin sensitivity and decrease blood sugar levels has been investigated. It can be added to various dishes and beverages for flavor without adding extra calories.

Legumes:

Beans, lentils, and chickpeas are high in fiber and protein, making them excellent choices for managing blood sugar levels. Additionally, their glycemic index is low.

Avocado:

Monounsaturated lipids, which are heart-healthy fats, are abundant in avocados. They also provide fiber and essential nutrients. While they are calorie-dense, their nutrient profile makes them a good choice in moderation.

Turmeric:

Curcumin, the active compound in turmeric, has anti-inflammatory properties and may help improve insulin sensitivity. Consider adding turmeric to your meals or enjoying it in the form of turmeric tea.

It's essential to focus on a well-rounded diet, portion control, and regular physical activity in addition to incorporating these superfoods into your meals. Additionally, individual responses to foods can vary, so it's advisable to consult with a healthcare professional or a registered dietitian to create a personalized nutrition plan tailored to your specific needs and preferences.

Whole Grains and Fiber-Rich Foods

Whole grains and fiber-rich foods play a crucial role in managing type 2 diabetes by contributing to better blood sugar control, improved satiety, and overall cardiovascular health. Here's why they are considered essential nutrients in the context of type 2 diabetes:

Complex Carbohydrates:

Whole grains are rich in complex carbohydrates. Unlike refined carbohydrates, which can cause rapid spikes in blood sugar levels, the complex carbohydrates in whole grains are broken down more slowly, leading to a gradual and steady rise in blood glucose. This helps in better blood sugar management for individuals with type 2 diabetes.

Fiber Content:

Fiber is a key component of whole grains and other plant-based foods. Dietary fiber comes in two primary varieties: soluble and insoluble. Both types offer health benefits for individuals with diabetes.

Soluble Fiber: Found in foods like oats, barley, legumes, and certain fruits, soluble fiber forms a gel-like substance in the digestive tract that can help slow down the absorption of glucose, leading to better blood sugar control.

Insoluble Fiber: Found in the outer layers of grains, vegetables, and whole fruits, insoluble fiber adds bulk to the stool and helps prevent constipation, a common issue for people with diabetes.

Satiety and Weight Management:

Foods rich in fiber are generally more filling and can contribute to a sense of satiety. This can be particularly beneficial for individuals with type 2 diabetes who are working on weight management, as maintaining a healthy weight is important for insulin sensitivity.

Heart Health:

Whole grains have been associated with improved cardiovascular health. Individuals with type 2 diabetes are at an increased risk of heart disease, so including heart-healthy foods in their diet is essential. The fiber, vitamins, and minerals in whole grains contribute to overall cardiovascular well-being.

Lower Glycemic Index:

Whole grains typically have a lower glycemic index compared to refined grains. In other words, their effect on blood sugar levels is smaller and occurs more gradually. Choosing whole grains can help stabilize blood glucose levels and reduce the risk of sudden spikes and crashes.

Examples of whole grains and fiber-rich foods that can be beneficial for individuals with type 2 diabetes include:

Brown rice

Quinoa

Whole wheat

Oats and oat bran

Barley

Legumes (beans, lentils, chickpeas)

Vegetables and fruits with high fiber content

It's important to note that while whole grains and fiber-rich foods are valuable components of a diabetes-friendly diet, overall dietary choices, portion control, and regular physical activity are integral parts of managing type 2 diabetes effectively. As always, individual dietary recommendations should be tailored to specific health needs and goals, and consulting with a healthcare professional or registered dietitian is advisable for personalized guidance.

Lean Proteins and Healthy Fats

In managing type 2 diabetes, incorporating lean proteins and healthy fats into your diet is important for overall health, blood sugar control, and weight management. Here's why lean proteins and healthy fats are beneficial and some examples of foods that fall into these categories:

Lean Proteins:

Blood Sugar Control:

Meals high in protein have less of an effect on blood sugar levels than meals high in carbs. Including lean proteins in meals can help stabilize blood glucose levels, preventing sharp spikes and providing a more sustained release of energy.

Satiety and Weight Management:

Protein is well known for its ability to satisfy hunger and keep you feeling fuller for longer.. This can be particularly beneficial for individuals with type 2 diabetes who are working on weight management, as maintaining a healthy weight can improve insulin sensitivity.

Muscle Health:

Adequate protein intake is crucial for maintaining muscle mass, which is important for overall metabolic health. It also supports tissue repair and immune function.

Sources of Lean Proteins:

Fish: Salmon, trout, mackerel, and other fatty fish rich in omega-3 fatty acids.

Poultry: Skinless chicken or turkey breast.

Meats that are lean, such as sirloin or pork loin

Plant-based proteins: Tofu, tempeh, legumes (beans, lentils, chickpeas), and edamame.

Healthy Fats:

Heart Health:

Heart health benefits from heart-healthy fats including polyunsaturated and monounsaturated fats. People with diabetes are at an increased risk of cardiovascular issues, so including these fats in the diet can help manage overall cardiovascular risk.

Blood Sugar Regulation:

Blood sugar levels can rise more gradually as a result of healthy fats' ability to slow down the absorption of carbohydrates. This can be particularly helpful in managing post-meal glucose levels.

Satiety:

Like proteins, fats contribute to a feeling of fullness. Including healthy fats in meals can help control appetite and reduce the likelihood of overeating.

Sources of Healthy Fats:

Avocado: Rich in monounsaturated fats and fiber.

Nuts and seeds: Almonds, walnuts, chia seeds, flaxseeds, and sunflower seeds.

One excellent source of monounsaturated fat is olive oil.

Fatty fish: Salmon, mackerel, and sardines, which provide omega-3 fatty acids.

Nut butters: Almond or natural peanut butter.

It's essential to focus on the quality and balance of your overall diet. Strive for a combination of lean proteins, healthy fats, whole grains, and plenty of vegetables and fruits. Portion control and choosing nutrient-dense foods are key components of a well-rounded diet for managing type 2 diabetes. As always, individual dietary recommendations should be tailored to specific health needs and goals, and consulting with a healthcare professional or registered dietitian is advisable for personalized guidance.

Fruits and Vegetables

In the management of type 2 diabetes, incorporating a variety of fruits and vegetables into your diet is important for several reasons. Fruits and vegetables are rich in essential nutrients, fiber, and antioxidants, which can contribute to overall health and help control blood sugar levels. Here are some key points about the role of fruits and vegetables in type 2 diabetes:

1. Nutrient Density:

Fruits and vegetables are nutrient-dense, meaning they provide a significant amount of vitamins, minerals, and antioxidants relative to their calorie content. This makes them an excellent choice for individuals with diabetes who need to manage their weight and overall nutrient intake.

2. Fiber Content:

Dietary fiber content is high in fruits and veggies alike. Fiber has multiple benefits for people with type 2 diabetes, including slowing down the absorption of glucose, improving insulin sensitivity, and aiding in weight management. Aim for a variety of colorful fruits and non-starchy vegetables to maximize your fiber intake.

3. Low Glycemic Index:

Many fruits and non-starchy vegetables have a low glycemic index (GI), which means they have a smaller impact on blood sugar levels. Examples of low-GI fruits include berries, cherries, and apples.Broccoli, cauliflower, and leafy greens are examples of non-starchy veggies that are ideal options.

4. Antioxidants:

Fruits and vegetables are rich in antioxidants, which help protect cells from damage caused by free radicals. This is particularly important for individuals with diabetes, as oxidative stress is linked to complications associated with the condition.

5. Portion Control:

While fruits are nutritious, it's important to be mindful of portion sizes, especially for those with diabetes. Opt for whole fruits rather than fruit juices, and spread fruit consumption throughout the day to avoid spikes in blood sugar.

6. Variety is Key:

Aim for a diverse range of fruits and vegetables to ensure you're getting a broad spectrum of nutrients. Include a mix of colors, as different colors often indicate different types of beneficial compounds.

7. Cooking Methods:

Choose healthy cooking methods, such as steaming, roasting, or sautéing, to preserve the nutritional content of fruits and vegetables. Avoid adding excessive amounts of unhealthy fats, sugars, or salt.

Examples of Diabetes-Friendly Fruits:

Berries (strawberries, blueberries, raspberries)

Apples

Cherries

Pears

Citrus fruits (oranges, grapefruits)

Examples of Diabetes-Friendly Vegetables:

Leafy greens (spinach, kale, Swiss chard)

Broccoli

Cauliflower

Bell peppers

Zucchini

It's important to individualize your diet based on factors such as personal preferences, cultural considerations, and any other health conditions you may have. Consulting with a healthcare professional or a registered dietitian can help you create a personalized and sustainable nutrition plan tailored to your specific needs and goals.

Foods to Avoid: High-Sugar Foods

For individuals with type 2 diabetes, managing blood sugar levels involves being mindful of their carbohydrate intake, especially when it comes to high-sugar foods. Here are some types of foods that are generally high in added sugars and may not be the best choices for those with type 2 diabetes:

Sugary Beverages:

Regular sodas, fruit juices, energy drinks, and sweetened teas can contain high amounts of added sugars. These drinks can lead to rapid spikes in blood sugar levels and contribute to weight gain.

Candies and Sweets:

Confections like candies, chocolates, cookies, cakes, pastries, and other sweet treats are typically high in sugars and should be limited. Opt for sugar-free or lower-sugar alternatives when possible.

Processed Snacks:

Many commercially available snacks, such as flavored granola bars, sugary cereals, and sweetened yogurt, can be high in added sugars. Check food labels for hidden sugars and choose snacks with lower sugar content.

Sweetened Breakfast Cereals:

Breakfast cereals with added sugars can contribute to a quick rise in blood sugar levels. Choose whole-grain, low-sugar cereals or oatmeal instead.

Flavored Yogurts:

Flavored yogurts often contain added sugars for flavor. Opt for plain, unsweetened yogurt and add fresh fruits or a small amount of honey for sweetness.

Desserts and Ice Cream:

Ice cream, pies, cakes, and other desserts are usually high in sugar and should be consumed in moderation. Consider healthier dessert alternatives, such as fruit salads or yogurt with berries.

Sweetened Condiments:

Condiments like ketchup, barbecue sauce, and some salad dressings can be high in added sugars. Look for low-sugar or sugar-free alternatives, and consider making your own dressings using olive oil and vinegar.

Processed Foods:

Many processed foods, including certain canned soups, sauces, and pre-packaged meals, can contain hidden sugars. Check food labels for added sugars and choose minimally processed options.

Dried Fruits:

While fruits are generally healthy, dried fruits can be concentrated sources of sugar. It's easy to consume larger portions of dried fruits, so be mindful of your intake.

Sports Drinks:

Sports drinks often contain added sugars and are designed for individuals engaged in intense physical activity. For hydration, water is a better choice for those with type 2 diabetes.

It's important to read food labels carefully to identify hidden sugars, as they can be listed under various names (e.g., sucrose, high-fructose corn syrup, agave nectar). Additionally, focusing on whole, unprocessed foods and emphasizing a well-balanced diet with lean proteins, healthy fats, and fiber-rich carbohydrates can contribute to better blood sugar control. If you have specific dietary concerns or questions, it's advisable to consult with a healthcare professional or a registered dietitian for personalized guidance.

Processed and Refined Carbohydrates

Processed and refined carbohydrates can have a significant impact on blood sugar levels and overall health, making them important to monitor and limit for individuals with type 2 diabetes. Here's why processed and refined carbohydrates can be problematic and some examples of foods to avoid:

1. Rapid Blood Sugar Spikes:

Processed and refined carbohydrates are often quickly digested and absorbed, leading to rapid spikes in blood sugar levels. This can challenge the body's ability to produce enough insulin to manage the increased glucose in the bloodstream.

2. Low Nutrient Density:

Many processed and refined carbohydrate sources lack essential nutrients, such as fiber, vitamins, and minerals. Consuming foods with low nutrient density can contribute to nutritional deficiencies and may not support overall health.

3. Limited Satiety:

Refined carbohydrates often lack the fiber and protein found in whole, unprocessed foods. As a result, they may not provide a sense of fullness or satiety, potentially leading to overeating and weight gain.

4. Increased Insulin Resistance:

Regular consumption of processed and refined carbohydrates may contribute to insulin resistance over time.One of the main contributing factors to the onset and course of type 2 diabetes is insulin resistance.

5. Risk of Weight Gain:

Diets high in processed and refined carbohydrates are associated with weight gain and obesity, which are risk factors for the development and management of type 2 diabetes.

Examples of Processed and Refined Carbohydrates to Limit:

White Bread and Pastries:

White bread, bagels, croissants, and other refined flour products can lead to rapid increases in blood sugar levels.

Sugary Breakfast Cereals:

Refined grains and added sugars are common ingredients in morning cereals. Opt for whole-grain, low-sugar options instead.

Sweetened Beverages:

Regular sodas, fruit juices, energy drinks, and sweetened teas are high in added sugars and can contribute to elevated blood sugar levels.

Packaged Snack Foods:

Chips, crackers, and other packaged snacks often contain refined carbohydrates and may be high in unhealthy fats and salt.

Instant or Flavored Rice and Pasta:

Instant rice, flavored rice mixes, and certain pasta products can be high in refined carbohydrates. Choose whole grains like brown rice and whole wheat pasta instead.

Processed Sweets and Desserts:

Cookies, cakes, candies, and other desserts made with refined sugars and flours should be limited.

Sweetened Yogurts:

Flavored yogurts often contain added sugars. To add natural sweetness, add fresh fruits to plain, unsweetened yogurt.

Commercially Baked Goods:

Commercially baked goods like muffins, doughnuts, and pastries are typically high in refined carbohydrates and sugars.

Healthy Alternatives:

Choose whole, unprocessed grains such as brown rice, quinoa, and oats.

Include a variety of colorful fruits and vegetables for fiber and essential nutrients.

Opt for whole-grain bread, pasta, and cereals with minimal added sugars.

Use sweeteners like honey or maple syrup in moderation, if necessary.

By focusing on whole, minimally processed foods and paying attention to portion sizes, individuals with type 2 diabetes can better manage their blood sugar levels and support overall health. As always, personalized dietary advice from a healthcare professional or registered dietitian is recommended.

Saturated and Trans Fats

Saturated fats and trans fats are types of dietary fats that can impact cardiovascular health and may have implications for individuals with type 2 diabetes. It's important for individuals with diabetes to be mindful of their fat intake, as certain types of fats can influence insulin sensitivity and overall heart health. Here's a breakdown of saturated and trans fats and their relevance to type 2 diabetes:

1. Saturated Fats:

Sources: Saturated fats are primarily found in animal products such as fatty cuts of meat, poultry with skin, full-fat dairy products, butter, and lard. Some plant-based sources, like coconut oil and palm oil, also contain saturated fats.

Impact on Health: High intake of saturated fats has been associated with an increased risk of cardiovascular disease, which is a significant concern for individuals with type 2 diabetes who are already at higher risk for heart-related complications.

Recommendations: While it's not necessary to eliminate saturated fats entirely, it's advisable to limit their intake. Choose lean cuts of meat, poultry without skin, and opt for low-fat or fat-free dairy products. Replace saturated fats with healthier options like mono- and polyunsaturated fats.

2. Trans Fats:

Sources: Trans fats are artificially created fats through a process called hydrogenation, which turns liquid oils into solid fats. They are commonly found in partially hydrogenated oils used in some processed and packaged foods, fried foods, and certain baked goods.

Impact on Health: Trans fats have been linked to an increased risk of cardiovascular disease, inflammation, and insulin resistance. They also tend to raise "bad" LDL cholesterol while lowering "good" HDL cholesterol.

Recommendations: Health authorities recommend minimizing trans fat intake as much as possible. Food labels may list 0 grams of trans fats if the content is below a certain threshold, so it's essential to check for partially hydrogenated oils in the ingredients list.

Dietary Recommendations for Individuals with Type 2 Diabetes:

Prioritize Healthy Fats: Choose sources of healthy fats, such as avocados, nuts, seeds, and olive oil. These fats, particularly monounsaturated and polyunsaturated fats, can have positive effects on heart health.

Limit Saturated Fats: Reduce the intake of saturated fats by choosing lean protein sources, opting for low-fat or fat-free dairy products, and using healthier cooking oils.

Avoid Trans Fats: Check food labels for the presence of partially hydrogenated oils, which indicate the presence of trans fats. Avoid or limit the consumption of foods containing trans fats.

Maintaining a balanced and heart-healthy diet is crucial for individuals with type 2 diabetes. This includes not only monitoring carbohydrate intake but also being mindful of the types and amounts of fats consumed. Consulting with a healthcare professional or a registered dietitian can provide personalized guidance on dietary choices that align with individual health needs and goals.

Sodium and High-Salt Foods

Sodium, a component of salt, is a mineral that is essential for various bodily functions. However, excessive sodium intake, often associated with a high-salt diet, can contribute to health issues, particularly for individuals with type 2 diabetes. Here's how sodium and high-salt foods can affect individuals with type 2 diabetes:

1. Blood Pressure and Cardiovascular Health:

High sodium intake is a known contributor to high blood pressure (hypertension). Individuals with type 2 diabetes are already at an increased risk of cardiovascular complications, and hypertension further elevates this risk. Managing blood pressure is crucial for overall heart health.

2. Fluid Retention:

Excessive sodium intake can lead to fluid retention, which may result in swelling and increased blood volume. This, in turn, can contribute to elevated blood pressure and strain on the cardiovascular system.

3. Kidney Health:

Diabetes is a leading cause of kidney disease, and high sodium intake can exacerbate kidney-related issues. The kidneys play a crucial role in regulating sodium balance in the body, and excessive sodium can contribute to kidney damage over time.

4. Increased Thirst and Urination:

High sodium levels can contribute to dehydration, leading to increased thirst and urination. Individuals with diabetes are already at risk for dehydration due to elevated blood sugar levels, and excessive sodium intake can further contribute to this risk.

5. Recommendations for Sodium Intake:
Health authorities, including the American Diabetes Association, recommend limiting sodium intake to promote heart health. The general guideline for sodium intake is to aim for less than 2,300 milligrams per day for most adults. However, those with diabetes, hypertension, or other cardiovascular issues may benefit from further reducing their sodium intake to 1,500 milligrams per day or as advised by healthcare professionals.

High-Salt Foods to Limit:

Processed and Packaged Foods: Many processed and packaged foods, including snacks, canned soups, and ready-made meals, can be high in sodium.

Fast Food: Fast food and restaurant meals can often contain excessive amounts of salt.

Deli Meats and Processed Meats: These can be high in sodium, so it's advisable to choose low-sodium or fresh alternatives.

Condiments and Sauces: Some condiments, sauces, and salad dressings can be sources of hidden sodium. Choose low-sodium alternatives or make your own.

Canned Vegetables and Beans: While convenient, canned vegetables and beans can have added salt. Rinsing them before use can help reduce sodium content.

Tips for Reducing Sodium Intake:

Choose fresh, whole foods over processed options.

Spices, herbs, and other flavorings can be used to improve food without adding salt.

Be mindful of portion sizes, as larger portions may contribute to higher sodium intake.
Check food labels for sodium content and choose lower-sodium alternatives.
Managing sodium intake is an essential component of a heart-healthy diet for individuals with type 2 diabetes. It's advisable to work with healthcare professionals or registered dietitians to create a personalized nutrition plan that considers individual health needs and dietary preferences

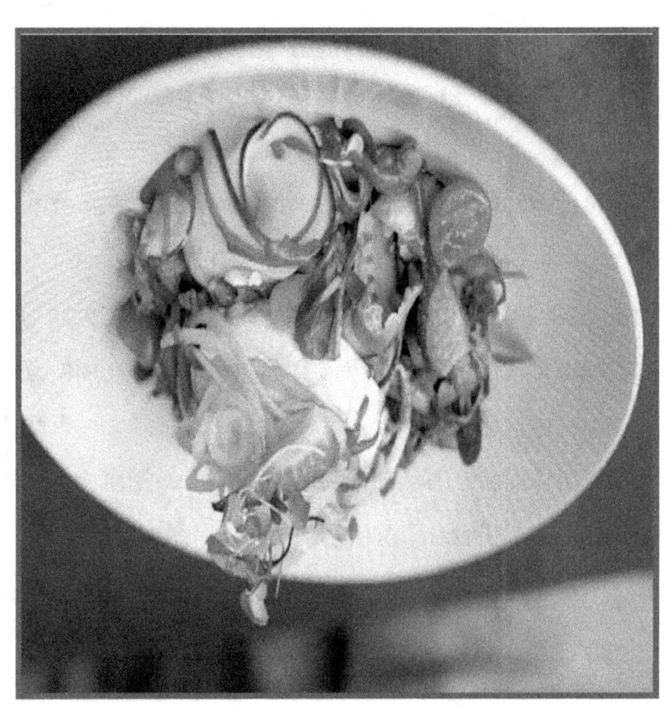

CHAPTER SIX: Meal Planning and Recipes

Creating Balanced Meals

Managing type 2 diabetes involves making healthy food choices to control blood sugar levels. Creating balanced meals that include a mix of carbohydrates, proteins, and fats is crucial. Here are detailed tips for creating balanced meals in type 2 diabetes management:

1. Carbohydrates:

Choose Complex Carbs: Opt for whole grains, legumes, vegetables, and fruits with low glycemic index (GI). These foods release glucose slowly, preventing rapid spikes in blood sugar.

Portion Control: To control your consumption of carbohydrates, pay attention to portion sizes. Use measuring tools to ensure accuracy.

Fiber-Rich Foods: Include high-fiber foods like vegetables, fruits, nuts, seeds, and whole grains. Fiber helps stabilize blood sugar levels and promotes satiety.

2. Proteins:

Lean Protein Sources: Include low-fat dairy, fish, chicken, tofu, and legumes in your diet. These proteins don't contribute to blood sugar spikes and aid in muscle maintenance.

Protein Distribution: Spread protein intake throughout the day to help control blood sugar levels and maintain muscle mass.

3. Fats:

Healthy Fats: Opt for foods high in avocados, nuts, seeds, and olive oil, among other healthy fat sources. Limit saturated and trans fats, found in processed foods and fatty cuts of meat.

Portion Control: While healthy fats are beneficial, they are calorie-dense. Control portions to manage overall calorie intake.

4. Meal Timing:

Regular Meals: Eat at consistent times each day to help regulate blood sugar levels. Avoid skipping meals to prevent overeating later.

Snacking: If needed, opt for healthy snacks like raw vegetables, nuts, or Greek yogurt between meals to maintain stable blood sugar levels.

5. Vegetables:

Colorful Variety: Include a variety of colorful vegetables to ensure a broad spectrum of nutrients. Non-starchy vegetables are particularly low in carbohydrates and high in fiber.

Cooking Methods: Opt for steaming, roasting, or sautéing instead of frying to retain the nutritional value of vegetables.

6. Beverages:

Hydration: To stay hydrated, sip lots of water throughout the day. Limit sugary beverages and opt for herbal tea, water, or infused water.

Alcohol Moderation: If you consume alcohol, do so in moderation and be aware of its impact on blood sugar levels.

7. Monitoring and Adaptation:

Frequent Monitoring: To learn how different foods influence you, monitor your blood sugar levels on a frequent basis.

Speak with a Dietitian: Create a customized meal plan with the help of a trained dietician that takes into account your tastes and requirements.

8. Physical Activity:

Regular Exercise: Include regular physical activity in your routine, as it helps improve insulin sensitivity and manage blood sugar levels.

9. Mindful Eating:

Slow and Mindful: Eat slowly, savoring each bite. This helps control portion sizes and promotes better digestion.

10. Individualized Approach:

Personalized Meal Plan: Work with healthcare professionals to create a meal plan tailored to your individual needs, considering factors like age, weight, activity level, and overall health.

Remember, these tips provide general guidance, and it's crucial to consult with healthcare professionals, especially a registered dietitian or nutritionist, for personalized advice based on your specific health conditions and requirements.

Sample Meal Plans

Creating a sample meal plan for type 2 diabetes involves incorporating a balance of carbohydrates, proteins, and fats while considering portion sizes. Keep in mind that individual needs vary, so it's crucial to customize these plans based on personal preferences, nutritional requirements, and any dietary restrictions. For individualized guidance, speak with a qualified dietitian or other medical practitioner. Here are three sample meal plans:

Sample Meal Plan 1:

Breakfast:

Scrambled eggs with spinach and tomatoes

Whole-grain toast

1 small apple

Black coffee or herbal tea

Lunch:

Grilled chicken breast

Quinoa or brown rice

Steamed broccoli and carrots

Mixed green salad with vinaigrette dressing

Snack:

Greek yogurt with a handful of mixed berries

Handful of almonds or walnuts

Dinner:

Baked salmon

Sweet potato wedges

Asparagus spears

Mixed salad with olive oil dressing

Snack (if needed):

Sliced cucumber with hummus

Sample Meal Plan 2:

Breakfast:

Strawberries cut into slices and a tablespoon of chia seeds added to oatmeal

Greek yogurt

Green tea or black coffee

Lunch:

Lentil and vegetable soup

Whole-grain roll

Mixed vegetable salad with a light vinaigrette dressing

Snack:

Cottage cheese with pineapple chunks

Handful of cherry tomatoes

Dinner:

Grilled turkey burger (or veggie burger)

Quinoa or cauliflower rice

Steamed green beans

Side salad with avocado

Snack (if needed):

A small pear with a handful of almonds

Sample Meal Plan 3:

Breakfast:

Smoothie with spinach, banana, berries, Greek yogurt, and a tablespoon of flaxseeds

Whole-grain English muffin

Lunch:

Stir-fried tofu with mixed vegetables (bell peppers, broccoli, and snap peas)

Brown rice

Side of sliced cucumbers

Snack:

Celery sticks with peanut butter

Small orange

Dinner:

Baked cod fillet

Quinoa pilaf with mixed herbs

Roasted Brussels sprouts and carrots

Side salad with balsamic vinaigrette

Snack (if needed):

A handful of mixed nuts and seeds

General Tips:

Hydration: Drink plenty of water throughout the day.

Portion Control: To control calorie consumption, pay attention to portion sizes.

Consistency: Aim for consistent meal timings and spacing throughout the day.

Monitor Blood Sugar Levels: Regularly monitor blood sugar levels to understand how different meals affect your body.

Remember, these sample meal plans are just examples, and individual nutritional needs may vary. It's important to work with healthcare professionals, especially a registered dietitian, to tailor a meal plan that meets your specific requirements and health goals.

Healthy Recipes for Type 2 Diabetes

Here are a few healthy recipes suitable for individuals with type 2 diabetes. Remember to consult with a healthcare professional or a registered dietitian to ensure that these recipes align with your specific dietary needs and health goals.

1. Grilled Salmon with Lemon and Herbs:

Ingredients:

4 salmon fillets (about 6 ounces each)

2 tablespoons olive oil

2 cloves garlic, minced

1 teaspoon dried thyme

1 teaspoon dried rosemary

Salt and pepper to taste

Lemon wedges for serving

Instructions:

Preheat the grill to medium-high heat.

In a small bowl, mix together olive oil, minced garlic, thyme, rosemary, salt, and pepper.

Brush the salmon fillets with the herb mixture on both sides.

Grill the salmon for about 4-5 minutes per side or until the fish flakes easily with a fork.

Serve with lemon wedges.

2. Quinoa and Black Bean Salad:

Ingredients:

1 cup quinoa, rinsed

2 cups water or low-sodium vegetable broth

1 can (15 oz) black beans, drained and rinsed

1 cup cherry tomatoes, halved

1 cup cucumber, diced

1/4 cup red onion, finely chopped

1/4 cup fresh cilantro, chopped

2 tablespoons olive oil

2 tablespoons lime juice

Salt and pepper to taste

Instructions:

Cook quinoa according to package instructions using water or low-sodium vegetable broth.

In a large bowl, combine cooked quinoa, black beans, cherry tomatoes, cucumber, red onion, and cilantro.

In a small bowl, whisk together olive oil, lime juice, salt, and pepper. After adding the dressing to the salad, toss to mix.

Let it cool for a minimum of half an hour before serving.

3. Chicken and Vegetable Stir-Fry:

Ingredients:

1 lb boneless, skinless chicken breast, thinly sliced

2 cups broccoli florets

1 bell pepper, thinly sliced

1 cup snap peas, ends trimmed

2 tablespoons low-sodium soy sauce

1 tablespoon sesame oil

1 tablespoon rice vinegar

1 tablespoon ginger, minced

2 cloves garlic, minced

1 tablespoon olive oil

Instructions:

In a bowl, mix soy sauce, sesame oil, rice vinegar, ginger, and garlic to make the sauce.

Heat olive oil in a wok or large skillet over medium-high heat.

Cook the chicken slices until they are thoroughly done and browned.

To the skillet, add the bell pepper, snap peas, and broccoli. Stir-fry the vegetables for 3–4 minutes, or until they are crisp-tender.

Pour the sauce over the chicken and vegetables, tossing to coat evenly.

Cook for a further two to three minutes, or until well heated.

Serve over brown rice or cauliflower rice.

4. Roasted Vegetable and Chickpea Salad:

Ingredients:

1 can (15 oz) of rinsed and drained chickpeas

2 cups cherry tomatoes, halved

1 zucchini, sliced

1 red onion, sliced

1 bell pepper, sliced

2 tablespoons olive oil

1 teaspoon dried oregano

1 teaspoon smoked paprika

Salt and pepper to taste

Fresh basil leaves for garnish

Instructions:

Preheat the oven to 400°F (200°C).

In a large bowl, toss chickpeas, cherry tomatoes, zucchini, red onion, and bell pepper with olive oil, oregano, smoked paprika, salt, and pepper.

Spread the mixture on a baking sheet in a single layer.

Roast in the oven for 25-30 minutes or until the vegetables are tender and slightly caramelized.

Garnish with fresh basil leaves before serving.

These recipes incorporate lean proteins, whole grains, and plenty of vegetables to provide a balanced and nutritious meal. Depending on your dietary needs and tastes, change the ingredients and portion sizes.

CHAPTER SEVEN: Medications, Insulin, and Treatment Management

Oral Medications

Often, doctors will prescribe oral drugs to assist regulate blood sugar levels. It's important to note that the information provided here is for general educational purposes, and individualized advice should be sought from a healthcare professional. Here are some key points about oral medications for type 2 diabetes:

Types of Oral Medications:

Metformin: This is usually the first-line medication. It helps reduce glucose production in the liver and improves the body's response to insulin.

Sulfonylureas: These drugs encourage the pancreas to release more insulin. Common examples include glipizide and glyburide.

Meglitinides: Similar to sulfonylureas, meglitinides also stimulate insulin release, but they have a shorter duration of action. Repaglinide is an example.

DPP-4 Inhibitors: These drugs help lower blood sugar levels by preventing the breakdown of incretin hormones, which stimulate insulin release. Sitagliptin is one such medication.

SGLT2 Inhibitors: These medications work by preventing the reabsorption of glucose in the kidneys, leading to increased glucose excretion in the urine. Canagliflozin and dapagliflozin are examples.

Thiazolidinediones (TZDs): TZDs improve insulin sensitivity in the body. Pioglitazone is a commonly prescribed TZD.

Alpha-glucosidase Inhibitors: These drugs slow down the digestion and absorption of carbohydrates, helping to reduce post-meal spikes in blood sugar. Acarbose is an example.

Administration:

Most oral medications come in tablet or pill form.

It's important to take the medication exactly as prescribed by the healthcare provider.

Some medications may be taken with meals, while others may be taken before or after meals.

Potential Side Effects:

Side effects can vary depending on the medication. Common side effects may include gastrointestinal issues, such as nausea or diarrhea.

Some medications may have specific considerations, such as monitoring liver function with certain drugs.

Monitoring:

Regular blood sugar monitoring is crucial to assess the effectiveness of the medication.

Healthcare providers may also monitor other parameters like HbA1c, kidney function, and liver function regularly.

Lifestyle Changes:
Medication is often combined with lifestyle modifications, including a healthy diet, regular exercise, and weight management.

Consultation with Healthcare Provider:
Regular follow-up appointments with a healthcare provider are essential to adjust medications as needed and address any concerns or questions.
It's important for individuals with type 2 diabetes to have an open and ongoing dialogue with their healthcare team to ensure the most effective and personalized treatment plan.

Insulin Therapy

Insulin therapy is a treatment option for managing type 2 diabetes when other methods such as oral medications, lifestyle changes, and diet are insufficient in controlling blood sugar levels. While insulin therapy is often associated with type 1 diabetes, it is increasingly used in type 2 diabetes when oral medications alone are not effective.

Role of Insulin Therapy in Type 2 Diabetes:

Supplementing Insulin Levels:

In type 2 diabetes, the body may not produce enough insulin, or the insulin produced may not work effectively (insulin resistance). Insulin therapy provides the body with the insulin it needs to regulate blood sugar levels.

Controlling Blood Sugar Levels:

Insulin is a hormone that helps cells take in glucose from the bloodstream. By using insulin injections, individuals with type 2 diabetes can regulate their blood sugar levels more effectively.

Managing High Blood Sugar:

Insulin therapy is particularly useful when blood sugar levels are consistently elevated, and other medications or lifestyle changes are not providing adequate control.

Combination Therapy:

In some cases, insulin therapy may be used in combination with oral medications to achieve better glycemic control. This approach is often referred to as "intensification" of treatment.

Flexibility and Precision:

Insulin therapy allows for precise control over blood sugar levels, as the dosage can be adjusted based on individual needs, daily activities, and dietary intake.

Types of Insulin:

There are different types of insulin, classified based on their onset, peak, and duration of action. Rapid-acting insulin, short-acting insulin, intermediate-acting insulin, and long-acting insulin are some examples. The choice of insulin type and regimen depends on individual circumstances and lifestyle.

Delivery Methods:

Insulin can be injected using syringes, insulin pens, or insulin pumps. The method of delivery is often chosen based on individual preferences and needs.

Considerations for Insulin Therapy in Type 2 Diabetes:

Individualization:

Insulin therapy is highly individualized. The healthcare provider will determine the appropriate type of insulin, dosage, and timing based on factors such as blood sugar levels, lifestyle, and preferences.

Education:

Proper education and training are crucial for individuals starting insulin therapy. This includes learning how to administer insulin, understanding dosage adjustments, and recognizing the signs of hypoglycemia.

Monitoring:

Regular blood glucose monitoring is essential to adjust insulin dosage and ensure optimal control.

Lifestyle Management:

Insulin therapy should be complemented by a healthy lifestyle, including a balanced diet, regular exercise, and weight management.

It's important for individuals with type 2 diabetes to work closely with their healthcare team to determine the most suitable treatment plan, including the potential use of insulin therapy. Regular communication with healthcare providers helps in adjusting treatment strategies based on individual needs and responses to therapy.

Managing Medications and Lifestyle Changes

Managing medications and incorporating lifestyle changes are key components in effectively managing type 2 diabetes. A holistic approach that combines medication adherence with healthy lifestyle practices can help control blood sugar levels and improve overall well-being. Here are some strategies for managing medications and lifestyle changes in type 2 diabetes:

1. Medication Adherence:

Follow Prescribed Dosages: Take medications as prescribed by your healthcare provider. It's crucial to adhere to the recommended dosage and schedule.

Understand Medications: Know the names, purposes, and potential side effects of your medications. If you have any concerns or experience side effects, discuss them with your healthcare team.

Set Reminders: Use tools such as pill organizers or smartphone reminders to ensure you take your medications on time.

Regular Check-ins: Schedule regular follow-up appointments with your healthcare provider to assess the effectiveness of your medications and make any necessary adjustments.

2. Healthy Eating:

Balanced Diet: Focus on a balanced and nutritious diet. A range of fruits, vegetables, whole grains, lean meats, and healthy fats should be consumed..

Carbohydrate Management: Monitor carbohydrate intake and choose complex carbohydrates over simple sugars. This helps in better blood sugar control.

Portion Control: Be mindful of portion sizes to avoid overeating, which can impact blood sugar levels.

Regular Meal Timing: Aim for regular meal times to help regulate blood sugar levels throughout the day.

3. Regular Physical Activity:

Exercise Routine: Engage in regular physical activity, as it helps improve insulin sensitivity and can contribute to better blood sugar control.

Choose Activities You Enjoy: Find physical activities you enjoy to make it more sustainable. This could include walking, swimming, cycling, or other forms of exercise.

Consistency is Key: Strive for consistency in your exercise routine. Even short, regular sessions can have positive effects.

4. Weight Management:
Set Realistic Goals: If overweight, aim for gradual and sustainable weight loss.Blood sugar regulation can greatly benefit from even a small weight decrease.

Healthy Habits: Focus on adopting healthy habits rather than extreme diets. Long-term, sustainable lifestyle modifications are more beneficial.

5. Stress Management:

Relaxation Techniques: Practice stress-reducing techniques such as meditation, deep breathing, or yoga. Blood sugar levels can be impacted by ongoing stress.

Adequate Sleep: Ensure you get sufficient, quality sleep. Lack of sleep can affect insulin sensitivity and overall health.

6. Regular Monitoring:

Blood Sugar Monitoring: Follow your healthcare provider's recommendations for regular blood sugar monitoring. This helps track the impact of lifestyle changes and medication on your diabetes management.

HbA1c Tests: Periodic HbA1c tests provide a longer-term view of your blood sugar control. Discuss the results with your healthcare team.

7. Open Communication:

Healthcare Team Collaboration: Keep an open line of communication with your healthcare team. Share any concerns, challenges, or changes in your health status.

Adjustments as Needed: Be prepared to make adjustments to your medication or lifestyle plan based on your healthcare provider's recommendations.

8. Education and Support:

Continuous Learning: Stay informed about diabetes management through reliable sources. Attend educational sessions or support groups if available.

Peer Support: Connect with others who have diabetes. Sharing experiences and tips can provide valuable insights and motivation.

Remember, the management of type 2 diabetes is a dynamic process that may require adjustments over time. A personalized approach that considers your individual needs, preferences, and health status is crucial. Regular communication with your healthcare team is key to achieving and maintaining effective diabetes management.

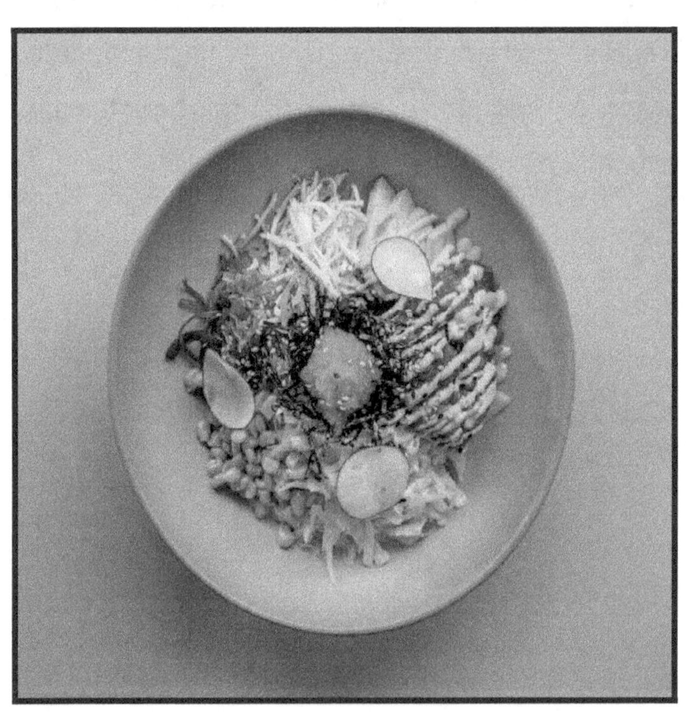

CHAPTER EIGHT: Potential Complications

Cardiovascular Complications

Type 2 diabetes is a chronic metabolic disorder characterized by insulin resistance and impaired insulin secretion. Individuals with type 2 diabetes are at an increased risk of developing cardiovascular complications. The cardiovascular complications associated with type 2 diabetes are a major cause of morbidity and mortality among affected individuals. Here are some key cardiovascular complications linked to type 2 diabetes:

Coronary Artery Disease (CAD): People with type 2 diabetes have a higher risk of developing coronary artery disease. Elevated blood glucose levels, insulin resistance, and other metabolic abnormalities contribute to the development of atherosclerosis, narrowing the coronary arteries and increasing the risk of heart attacks.

Myocardial Infarction (Heart Attack): Individuals with type 2 diabetes have an increased risk of myocardial infarction due to the accelerated development of atherosclerosis and the vulnerability of atherosclerotic plaques. Moreover, diabetes can affect the response to a heart attack, making recovery more challenging.

Stroke: Diabetes is a significant risk factor for ischemic stroke. The risk is attributed to factors such as atherosclerosis, hypertension, and the adverse effects of diabetes on blood vessels, including small vessel disease.

Peripheral Artery Disease (PAD): Diabetes increases the risk of peripheral artery disease, which is characterized by reduced blood flow to the extremities, often leading to pain, ulcers, and an increased risk of amputation.

Hypertension: Hypertension (high blood pressure) is a common comorbidity in individuals with type 2 diabetes. The combination of diabetes and hypertension significantly increases the risk of cardiovascular events.

Heart Failure: Diabetes is a risk factor for heart failure, and individuals with diabetes are more likely to develop heart failure even in the absence of coronary artery disease. Poorly controlled diabetes can lead to damage of the heart muscle, impairing its ability to pump blood effectively.

Dyslipidemia: Diabetes often leads to abnormal lipid profiles, including elevated levels of triglycerides and decreased levels of high-density lipoprotein (HDL) cholesterol. These lipid abnormalities contribute to the development of atherosclerosis.

Microvascular Complications: While not exclusive to the cardiovascular system, microvascular complications such as diabetic nephropathy (kidney disease) and retinopathy (eye disease) are common in individuals with type 2 diabetes and can indirectly impact cardiovascular health.

Management of type 2 diabetes involves lifestyle modifications, medications (including those targeting glucose control, blood pressure, and cholesterol levels), and regular monitoring to reduce the risk of cardiovascular complications. It is crucial for individuals with type 2 diabetes to work closely with healthcare professionals to control blood glucose levels and manage cardiovascular risk factors effectively. Regular check-ups, a healthy diet, regular physical activity, and medication adherence are essential components of a comprehensive diabetes management plan.

Neuropathy

Neuropathy is a common and potentially serious complication of type 2 diabetes. It refers to damage or dysfunction of the nerves, particularly those in the peripheral nervous system. The peripheral nervous system includes nerves outside the brain and spinal cord, responsible for transmitting signals between the central nervous system and the rest of the body, such as the limbs and organs.

In the context of type 2 diabetes, neuropathy is often classified into several types:

Peripheral Neuropathy: This is the most common type of neuropathy associated with diabetes. It typically affects the nerves of the feet and legs, but can also involve the hands and arms. Symptoms may include pain, tingling, numbness, and weakness in the affected areas. Peripheral neuropathy can lead to complications such as foot ulcers, infections, and difficulties with balance and coordination.

Autonomic Neuropathy: This type of neuropathy affects the autonomic nervous system, which controls involuntary functions such as heart rate, blood pressure, digestion, and bladder function. Symptoms can include gastrointestinal issues (such as gastroparesis), cardiovascular problems (such as heart rate abnormalities), and genitourinary symptoms.

Proximal Neuropathy: Also known as diabetic amyotrophy or radiculoplexus neuropathy, this type of neuropathy affects the hips, thighs, and buttocks. It can cause severe pain, muscle weakness, and difficulty moving the legs.

Focal Neuropathy: Focal neuropathy occurs when there is damage to a specific nerve or group of nerves, resulting in localized symptoms. It often affects the head, torso, or leg. Unlike other types of neuropathy, focal neuropathy can resolve on its own over time.

The exact mechanisms through which diabetes leads to neuropathy are not completely understood. However, prolonged exposure to high blood sugar levels is believed to play a significant role. Other contributing factors include inflammation, oxidative stress, and metabolic imbalances.

Preventing and managing neuropathy in type 2 diabetes involves maintaining good blood glucose control. Additionally, lifestyle modifications such as regular exercise, a healthy diet, and avoiding smoking can help reduce the risk of neuropathic complications. Medications may be prescribed to manage symptoms such as pain.

Regular monitoring and early intervention are crucial in managing diabetic neuropathy to prevent complications and improve the quality of life for individuals with type 2 diabetes. It's important for individuals with diabetes to work closely with healthcare professionals to develop a comprehensive care plan that addresses both blood glucose control and the prevention or management of complications like neuropathy.

Kidney Issues

Kidney issues, specifically diabetic nephropathy, are significant complications associated with type 2 diabetes. Diabetic nephropathy is a condition characterized by damage to the kidneys due to diabetes. Over time, high blood sugar levels can lead to structural and functional changes in the kidneys, impairing their ability to filter waste products and excess fluids from the blood. Here is a comprehensive overview of kidney issues in the context of type 2 diabetes:

Pathophysiology:

Glomerular Damage: The glomeruli, tiny blood vessels in the kidneys responsible for filtration, can be damaged by prolonged exposure to elevated glucose levels. This damage can lead to increased permeability and leakage of proteins into the urine.

Renal Hypertrophy: Diabetes can cause hypertrophy (enlargement) of the kidneys as they attempt to compensate for increased filtration demands. However, this enlargement is not beneficial and contributes to long-term damage.

Inflammation and Fibrosis: Chronic inflammation and the deposition of extracellular matrix proteins in the kidney tissues contribute to fibrosis, impairing kidney function.

Stages of Diabetic Nephropathy:

Diabetic nephropathy typically progresses through the following stages:

Microalbuminuria: Small amounts of albumin (a protein) leak into the urine.

Proteinuria: Increased levels of protein in the urine, indicating more severe kidney damage.

Reduced Glomerular Filtration Rate (GFR): The kidneys' ability to filter blood decreases, leading to waste accumulation in the body.

End-Stage Renal Disease (ESRD): The final stage where kidneys fail completely, requiring dialysis or kidney transplantation.

Risk Factors:

Poorly controlled blood glucose levels.

Hypertension (high blood pressure).

Genetic predisposition.

Smoking.

Elevated cholesterol levels.

Clinical Presentation:

Early Stages: Diabetic nephropathy may be asymptomatic in its early stages.

Later Stages: Symptoms may include fatigue, swelling (edema), difficulty concentrating, decreased appetite, and increased or decreased urine output.

Diagnosis:

Urinalysis: Detects the presence of proteins, especially albumin, in the urine.

Blood Tests: Measure serum creatinine and estimate GFR to assess kidney function.

Imaging: Ultrasound or other imaging techniques may be used to assess kidney structure.

Management and Prevention:

Blood Glucose Control: Tight glycemic control is crucial in preventing and managing diabetic nephropathy.

Blood Pressure Management: Controlling hypertension is essential in slowing the progression of kidney damage.

Medications: Angiotensin-converting enzyme (ACE) inhibitors and angiotensin II receptor blockers (ARBs) are commonly used to protect the kidneys.

Lifestyle Modifications: Healthy lifestyle choices, including a balanced diet, regular exercise, and avoiding smoking, can contribute to kidney health.

Regular Monitoring: Periodic monitoring of kidney function through blood and urine tests is essential for early detection and intervention.

Complications:

Cardiovascular complications are common in individuals with diabetic nephropathy.

Increased risk of fluid and electrolyte imbalances.

Anemia due to reduced production of erythropoietin by the kidneys

Diabetic nephropathy is a serious complication of type 2 diabetes that requires comprehensive management. Early detection, along with effective blood glucose and blood pressure control, can significantly slow the progression of kidney damage and reduce the risk of complications. Regular follow-ups with healthcare professionals are crucial for monitoring kidney function and adjusting treatment plans as needed.

Eye Complications

Type 2 diabetes can lead to various eye complications, collectively referred to as diabetic eye disease. These complications are primarily associated with damage to the small blood vessels in the retina, the light-sensitive tissue at the back of the eye. The most common diabetic eye complications include:

1. Diabetic Retinopathy:

Background Retinopathy: In the early stages, small bulges (microaneurysms) may form in the blood vessels of the retina.

Macular Edema: Fluid leakage from retinal blood vessels can lead to swelling of the macula, the central part of the retina responsible for sharp vision.

Proliferative Retinopathy: Advanced stage characterized by the growth of abnormal blood vessels on the surface of the retina, which can lead to bleeding and scarring.

2. Diabetic Macular Edema (DME):

Accumulation of fluid in the macula, causing it to swell. This can lead to blurred or distorted vision.

3. Cataracts:

People with diabetes are at an increased risk of developing cataracts, a clouding of the lens in the eye, leading to blurred vision.

4. Glaucoma:

Diabetes increases the risk of glaucoma, a condition characterized by increased pressure within the eye that can damage the optic nerve and lead to vision loss.

Risk Factors for Diabetic Eye Complications:

Poorly Controlled Blood Glucose Levels: Prolonged periods of high blood sugar contribute to the development and progression of eye complications.

Hypertension (High Blood Pressure): Elevated blood pressure can exacerbate diabetic eye disease.

Duration of Diabetes: The longer a person has diabetes, the higher the risk of developing eye complications.

Genetics: Family history may play a role in the susceptibility to diabetic eye disease.

Symptoms:

Blurred or Distorted Vision: Common in diabetic retinopathy and macular edema.

Floaters: Dark spots or strings in the field of vision, indicating bleeding or fluid leakage.

Poor Night Vision: Having trouble seeing in dimly lit areas.

Prevention and Management:

Regular Eye Exams: Annual comprehensive eye exams are crucial for early detection and intervention.

Blood Glucose Control: Tight glycemic control helps prevent and slow the progression of diabetic eye complications.

Blood Pressure Management: Controlling hypertension is essential in reducing the risk of eye problems.

Lifestyle Modifications: Healthy lifestyle choices, including a balanced diet, regular exercise, and avoiding smoking, can contribute to eye health.

Early Intervention: Prompt treatment of diabetic retinopathy or other eye issues can prevent or minimize vision loss

Diabetic eye complications are serious and can lead to significant vision impairment or blindness if not detected and managed early. Regular eye exams, along with comprehensive diabetes care, are essential for preventing, monitoring, and treating these complications. Individuals with type 2 diabetes should work closely with eye care professionals and healthcare providers to maintain optimal eye health and preserve vision.

CHAPTER NINE: Support and Community

Building a Support System

Building a support system for someone with type 2 diabetes is crucial for their well-being and long-term management of the condition. Here are some steps you can take to create an effective support system:

Educate Friends and Family:

Ensure that friends and family members are well-informed about type 2 diabetes. Share information about the condition, its management, and potential challenges. This will help them understand the individual's needs and provide appropriate support.

Encourage Healthy Lifestyle Changes:

Promote a healthy lifestyle for the person with diabetes and those around them. Encourage regular exercise, a balanced diet, and stress management. Making these changes together can foster a supportive environment and make it easier for the individual to adhere to their treatment plan.

Attend Medical Appointments Together:

Offer to accompany the person to medical appointments. This can provide emotional support, help with understanding medical advice, and allow you to discuss concerns with healthcare professionals.

Learn to Recognize Signs of Hypoglycemia:

Teach close contacts how to recognize the signs of low blood sugar (hypoglycemia) and what actions to take in case of an emergency. Quick response to hypoglycemia is essential for the person's safety.

Create a Healthy Home Environment:

Make the home a supportive environment by keeping healthy food options available, encouraging regular physical activity, and minimizing stress. This can positively impact the person's ability to manage their diabetes.

Emotional Support:

Diabetes management can be emotionally challengingBe present to offer emotional support and to listen. Encourage them to express their emotions and worries in an honest manner. Understanding that it's okay to have moments of frustration or anxiety can be comforting.

Join Support Groups:

Explore local or online diabetes support groups where the person can connect with others facing similar challenges. Sharing experiences and advice with people who understand the journey can be empowering and provide valuable insights.

Promote Medication Adherence:

Help the individual stay on track with their medication regimen. This may involve setting reminders, organizing pillboxes, or providing assistance when needed.

Encourage Regular Monitoring:

Support regular monitoring of blood glucose levels. Offer assistance with testing equipment, and celebrate achievements when blood sugar levels are well-managed.

Be Inclusive in Social Activities:

Include the person with diabetes in social activities that promote a healthy lifestyle. Whether it's going for a walk, cooking a healthy meal together, or engaging in other shared interests, inclusion fosters a sense of normalcy.

Remember that support is an ongoing process, and the needs of individuals with type 2 diabetes may change over time. Adapt and adjust your support system based on their evolving requirements.

Joining Diabetes Support Groups

Joining diabetes support groups can be a valuable and empowering step for individuals living with type 2 diabetes. These groups provide a supportive environment where members can share experiences, gain knowledge, and receive emotional encouragement. Here are some benefits and considerations of joining diabetes support groups:

Benefits:

Emotional Support:

Diabetes can be emotionally challenging, and individuals may experience feelings of isolation or frustration. Joining a support group provides a safe space to express these emotions, receive empathy, and connect with others who understand the journey.

Information and Education:

Support groups often serve as a rich source of information. Members can share insights about managing diabetes, coping with challenges, and staying updated on the latest treatments and technologies. Learning from others' experiences can enhance one's own understanding of the condition.

Motivation and Inspiration:

Being part of a community that shares similar goals and struggles can be motivating. Hearing success stories, learning about others' achievements in managing their diabetes, and sharing personal milestones can inspire individuals to stay committed to their health goals.

Practical Tips and Strategies:

Support groups offer a platform for members to exchange practical tips and strategies for managing diabetes on a daily basis. This can include advice on meal planning, exercise routines, medication management, and dealing with specific challenges.

Reduced Feelings of Isolation:

Living with a chronic condition like type 2 diabetes can sometimes lead to feelings of isolation. Joining a support group helps individuals realize that they are not alone. Connecting with others who face similar challenges fosters a sense of community and belonging.

Improved Adherence to Treatment Plans:

The accountability and encouragement within a support group can positively impact an individual's adherence to their treatment plan.

Knowing that others share similar goals creates a sense of collective commitment to health.

Considerations:

Find the Right Fit:

Support groups vary in structure and focus. Some may be in-person meetings, while others may be online forums or social media groups. It's essential to find a group that aligns with personal preferences and needs.

Respect for Diverse Experiences:

Diabetes affects individuals differently, and experiences may vary. In a support group, it's crucial to approach discussions with an open mind, respecting the diverse perspectives and challenges faced by members.

Balancing Online and In-Person Interaction:

Online support groups offer convenience, especially for those with busy schedules or limited mobility. However, in-person meetings can provide a more personal connection. Consider a combination of both to maximize the benefits.

Confidentiality and Privacy:

Ensure that the support group prioritizes confidentiality and respects members' privacy. A safe and trusting environment is essential for open and honest discussions.

Professional Guidance:

While support groups offer valuable peer support, they are not a substitute for professional medical advice. It's important to continue consulting healthcare professionals for personalized guidance on diabetes management.

Joining a diabetes support group can be a positive and enriching experience for individuals with type 2 diabetes. It not only provides valuable insights into managing the condition but also fosters a sense of community and mutual support that can enhance overall well-being.

Mental Health and Coping Strategies

Mental health is a crucial aspect of overall well-being, and it plays a significant role in the management of type 2 diabetes. Individuals living with diabetes often face unique challenges that can impact their mental health. It's essential to address these challenges and implement coping strategies to promote a positive mindset and effective diabetes management. Here are some insights into mental health considerations and coping strategies for individuals with type 2 diabetes:

Mental Health Considerations:

Emotional Impact:

The daily management of type 2 diabetes, including monitoring blood glucose levels, adhering to treatment plans, and making lifestyle changes, can be emotionally challenging. Anxiety, stress, and feelings of frustration may arise.

Fear of Complications:

Concerns about potential complications, such as cardiovascular issues, nerve damage, and kidney problems, can contribute to heightened anxiety. It's essential to address these fears and work towards preventive measures.

Social Impact:

Diabetes can sometimes lead to feelings of isolation, especially if individuals perceive a lack of understanding from others. Social situations may be affected, and managing diabetes in public settings can be a source of stress.

Body Image and Self-Esteem:

Changes in body weight, appearance, or the need for medication can impact body image and self-esteem. It's important to address these concerns and promote a positive self-image.

Coping Strategies:

Seek Professional Support:

Consider consulting with mental health professionals, such as psychologists or counselors, to address emotional challenges. Professionals can provide coping strategies and support tailored to the individual's needs.

Build a Strong Support System:

Surround yourself with a supportive network of friends, family, and peers who understand the challenges of living with diabetes. Open communication and sharing experiences can foster a sense of connection and understanding.

Practice Stress-Reducing Techniques:

Incorporate stress-reducing techniques into daily life, such as mindfulness, meditation, deep breathing exercises, or yoga. These practices can help manage stress levels and promote mental well-being.

Set Realistic Goals:

Establish achievable goals for diabetes management. Breaking down larger tasks into smaller, manageable steps can prevent feelings of overwhelm and increase a sense of accomplishment.

Stay Informed:

Knowledge is empowering. Stay informed about diabetes management, treatment options, and lifestyle changes. Understanding the condition can alleviate anxiety and contribute to a sense of control.

Regular Exercise:

Physical activity is not only beneficial for diabetes management but also for mental health.Frequent exercise releases endorphins, which have been shown to lessen stress and enhance happiness.

Healthy Lifestyle Choices:

Make positive lifestyle choices, including a balanced diet, regular sleep patterns, and adequate hydration. These factors contribute not only to physical health but also to mental well-being.

Join Support Groups:

As mentioned earlier, joining diabetes support groups can provide both practical advice and emotional support. Making connections with people who have gone through similar things might help fight feelings of loneliness.

Celebrate Achievements:

Acknowledge and celebrate personal achievements in diabetes management. Whether it's reaching a blood glucose target, maintaining a healthy lifestyle, or overcoming a challenge, recognizing success can boost self-esteem.

Regular Check-ins with Healthcare Professionals:

Schedule regular check-ups with healthcare professionals to monitor physical health and discuss any mental health concerns. A collaborative approach between healthcare providers and individuals with diabetes is crucial for comprehensive care.

Prioritizing mental health alongside physical health is integral for individuals living with type 2 diabetes. By implementing these coping strategies and seeking appropriate support, individuals can better navigate the challenges of diabetes while promoting overall well-being.

CHAPTER TEN: Success Stories

Real-life Experiences of Reversing Type 2 Diabetes

Real-life experiences of reversing type 2 diabetes are varied and can provide valuable insights into the potential for positive outcomes through lifestyle changes. While not everyone may achieve complete reversal, many individuals have reported significant improvements in their blood sugar levels, overall health, and quality of life by adopting healthier habits. It's essential to recognize that individual responses to interventions can vary, and any efforts to manage diabetes should be done in consultation with healthcare professionals. Here are some common themes seen in real-life experiences:

Dietary Changes:

Many individuals have successfully reversed or improved their type 2 diabetes by making significant changes to their diet. Adopting a low-carbohydrate, high-fiber diet, focusing on whole foods, and controlling portion sizes have been reported to be effective in managing blood sugar levels.

Weight Loss:

Weight loss is often associated with improvements in insulin sensitivity and blood glucose control. Real-life stories often highlight the positive impact of achieving and maintaining a healthy weight through a combination of diet and regular exercise.

Regular Exercise:

Incorporating regular physical activity into one's routine is a common thread in successful diabetes management. Exercise helps in weight management, improves insulin sensitivity, and contributes to overall cardiovascular health.

Monitoring Blood Sugar Levels:

Regular monitoring of blood sugar levels allows individuals to understand how different foods and activities affect their diabetes. This real-time feedback helps in making informed decisions about lifestyle choices.

Stress Management:

Stress can impact blood sugar levels, and.
under medical supervision.

Patient Advocacy:

Taking an active role in one's healthcare and being an advocate for personal well-being is a common theme. Real-life experiences often highlight the importance of being informed, asking questions, and working collaboratively with healthcare providers.

Community Support:

Support from friends, family, and diabetes support groups plays a significant role in the journey of managing and potentially reversing type 2 diabetes. Sharing experiences, challenges, and successes with others who understand the journey can be motivating and empowering.

Long-Term Commitment:

Reversing type 2 diabetes is often portrayed as a long-term commitment rather than a quick fix. Real-life stories emphasize the need for sustained lifestyle changes and ongoing vigilance in managing the condition.

It's crucial to approach discussions about reversing type 2 diabetes with a realistic perspective. Not everyone will experience complete reversal, and individual responses to interventions can vary. Furthermore, each person's health profile is unique, and what works for one individual may not work for another. Always consult with healthcare professionals before making significant changes to your diabetes management plan.

Tips and Insights from Those Who Have Success

Learning from the success stories of individuals who have effectively managed type 2 diabetes can provide valuable tips and insights. Here are some common tips derived from real-life experiences:

Commit to Lifestyle Changes:

Successful management often involves a commitment to long-term lifestyle changes. This includes adopting a balanced and nutritious diet, engaging in regular physical activity, and making sustainable adjustments to daily habits.

Educate Yourself:

Those who successfully manage type 2 diabetes often stress the importance of education. Understanding the condition, its implications, and the role of lifestyle choices can empower individuals to make informed decisions about their health.

Regular Monitoring:

Monitoring blood sugar levels regularly is a key aspect of successful diabetes management. It provides insights into how various factors, such as diet, exercise, and stress, affect blood glucose levels, allowing for timely adjustments.

Choose Whole Foods:

A common theme is the emphasis on whole, unprocessed foods. Adopting a diet rich in fruits, vegetables, lean proteins, and whole grains can contribute to better blood sugar control and overall health.

Portion Control:

Managing portion sizes is crucial for controlling blood sugar levels and supporting weight management. Real-life success stories often highlight the importance of portion control in meal planning.

Regular Exercise:

Incorporating regular physical activity is a consistent factor among those who successfully manage type 2 diabetes. Exercise improves insulin sensitivity, helps with weight management, and promotes overall well-being.

Customize Your Approach:

Recognize that there is no one-size-fits-all solution. Successful individuals often experiment with various lifestyle changes to find what works best for them, whether it's specific dietary patterns, exercise routines, or stress management techniques.

Consistency Matters:

Consistency in lifestyle choices is key. Establishing and maintaining a routine for meals, exercise, and medication (if prescribed) contributes to stable blood sugar levels over time.

Stay Hydrated:

Drinking an adequate amount of water is often mentioned as a simple yet important practice.

Proper hydration supports overall health and can contribute to better blood sugar control.

Seek Professional Guidance:

Successful diabetes management often involves collaboration with healthcare professionals. Regular check-ups, discussions about treatment plans, and adjustments based on medical advice contribute to positive outcomes.

Mindful Eating:

Practicing mindful eating, which involves paying attention to hunger and fullness cues, can help individuals make healthier food choices and avoid overeating.

Build a Support System:

Surrounding oneself with a supportive network, including friends, family, and healthcare professionals, is crucial. Sharing the journey with others who understand the challenges can provide emotional support and motivation.

Celebrate Small Victories:

Recognize and celebrate small achievements along the way. Whether it's reaching a weight loss goal, consistently hitting blood sugar targets, or adopting a new healthy habit, acknowledging progress is essential for motivation.

Manage Stress:

Stress management is highlighted by many as a critical aspect of diabetes care. Practices such as meditation, deep breathing, or engaging in hobbies can help reduce stress levels.

Remember, individual experiences may vary, and it's essential to tailor strategies to your specific needs and in consultation with healthcare professionals. Successful management of type 2 diabetes often involves a holistic and personalized approach.

CONCLUSION: A New Chapter Awaits

Congratulations on reaching the final page of "Reversing Type 2 Diabetes." As you close this chapter, we want you to carry with you the essence of empowerment, hope, and the knowledge that transformation is within your grasp.

Reflect on Your Journey

Take a moment to reflect on the insights gained, the stories shared, and the practical strategies unveiled. This isn't just a book; it's a roadmap to reclaiming control over your health. Whether you're just starting your journey or have implemented these changes into your life, remember that every step counts.

Your Health, Your Story

Your health is a narrative waiting to be written, and you now possess the pen. Each decision, each lifestyle change is a sentence that contributes to the plot of your health story. Embrace the power you hold and approach each day as an opportunity to shape a healthier, more vibrant future.

A Community of Support

You are not alone on this journey. Within these pages, you've discovered a community of individuals, like yourself, committed to reversing Type 2 Diabetes. Share your victories, seek guidance in challenges, and let the collective strength of this community propel you forward.

Stay Committed, Embrace Change

As you step away from this book, carry the commitment to yourself and your well-being. Embrace change as a friend, not a foe, and trust in the process. The journey to reversing Type 2 Diabetes is not without its twists and turns, but with determination and the knowledge gained, success is not only achievable but inevitable.

Your Next Chapter Begins Now
Your health journey doesn't end with the last page of this book; it's a continuous adventure. Implement what you've learned, be kind to yourself, and celebrate the progress, no matter how small. Your next chapter is filled with potential, vitality, and a life free from the constraints of Type 2 Diabetes.

Thank you for entrusting us with a part of your journey. We believe in your ability to create a healthier, happier future. Here's to the beginning of your new chapter!

Wishing you health, happiness, and boundless possibilities,

THANK YOU NOTE

Dear Esteemed Reader,

Thank you for embarking on the transformative journey through "Reversing Type 2 Diabetes." Your commitment to exploring new paths towards health and well-being is commendable, and we are thrilled to be a part of your quest for a diabetes-free life.

As you dive into the pages of this guide, know that your dedication to embracing change is the first step towards a brighter, healthier future. Your journey is unique, and we are grateful to have you on this path with us.

May the insights shared within these pages empower you, inspire you, and guide you towards a life filled with vitality and joy. Remember, each page turned is a step closer to rewriting your health story.

Thank you for choosing "Reversing Type 2 Diabetes." Here's to your health, happiness, and the limitless possibilities that await you.

With sincere gratitude,

Karla Mayer

[Author/Publisher]

9 798877 339156